ALSO BY CHICORO

in the Beautify Bit By Bit Series

Grow It! How to Grow Afro-Textured Hair to
Maximum Lengths in the Shortest Time

Beautify Bit By Bit

Hair Products 101

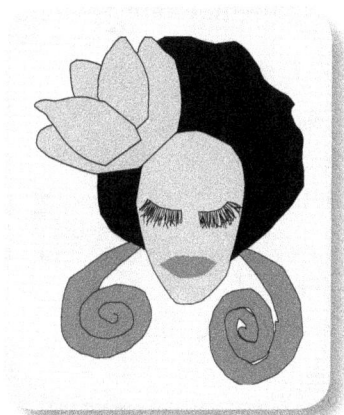

A 4-STEP PROCESS TO EMPOWER YOU TO SELECT THE BEST PRODUCTS FOR YOUR HAIR

Chicoro

Hair Care 101: A 4-Step Process to Empower You to Select the Best Products for Your Hair by Chicoro

ISBN: 978-09820689-2-2
Library of Congress Control Number: 2011911174

Printed in the United States of America

10 9 8 7 6 5 4 3 2 1

Published by ChicoroGYA Publishing
Web site: BeautifyBitByBitGi.com
E-mail: chicoro@beautifybitbybitgi.com

Photograph by Mark Oehler, www.mark-oehler.com
Cover Design by BookCoverExpress.com
Interior Design & Typesetting by Jill Ronsley, SunEditWrite.com

Disclaimer

The reader should use their own judgment in utilizing the information in this book. The author and publisher are not professional hair care providers, beauticians, dermatologists, hairstylists or cosmetologists. The reader should seek advice from professionals as needed.

The author's advice and information are based upon years of experience in trying to find a way to attain healthy, thick, long Afro-textured hair. This experience includes research done through studying books, taking classes and working with her own hair and that of other people.

This book is for educational and entertainment purposes. The publisher and author shall have neither responsibility nor liability to any person or entity with respect to any loss or damage alleged to be caused directly or indirectly by the advice or information contained herein.

Dedication

To all the beautiful, intelligent and caring women who have taken the time to write me their questions, comments and support. This book was born because of you. You showed me how to explain the process and put it in writing. I can't tell you how much I appreciate you. You all have taught me so much!

I wrote this book because it is humanly impossible for me to send an email to every person who wants a process that can help her pick hair care products. I hope some part of it will be helpful as you continue on your hair journey.

Acknowledgements

I would like to say thank you to the internationally renowned scientist and cosmetic chemist J. Alan Swift. It seems as though every article or book I found about hair mentioned the work of Dr. Swift. He was so generous as to buy my first book and provide feedback on it.

To Anthony L.L. Hunting, of Micelle Press, Inc., for his wonderful Cosmetic Encyclopedias of Shampoo and Conditioning Ingredients. These books are not only extremely informative, they are true works of art.

To Dallas Miller and Haven, for inspiring the cover image of this book. Swirling hair captured in a photograph is so beautiful. Thank you for showing me how it's done.

To Art West, for letting me talk him to death and test my ideas on him every day. Thank you for all the support and encouragement.

To my photographer, Mark Oehler, for making every woman he photographs, including me, look and feel beautiful, no matter how ordinary or plain she may look to the world. That's talent!

Finally, thank you to Virginia Milam, of Virginia's House of Beauty, who made sure that my locks were healthy and flowing. You are a great stylist. I appreciate your tremendous patience and gentleness. When I go to your shop to get my hair done, you always make me feel welcome and important. Lots of love and appreciation to you.

Table of Contents

CHAPTER 1

What This Book Is Not

This book focuses on store-bought products. It does not address the concoctions and formulas many of us make at home. The majority of the questions I receive are not about natural home-made products and ingredients. People's confusion relates more to store-bought products, and hence it is those products that are discussed in this book.

I am not going to tell you which brands of hair care products to buy and which ingredients are best for your hair. Many wonderful resources are available to do that. My goal is to help you understand the ingredients that are in the products. I believe that if you truly understand hair and hair care products, you will be able to decipher the information given and find those products that will work best for you. You will be able to make your own decisions.

It is up to you to determine whether certain ingredients are good or bad for you. It's not that I have a secret and am withholding information. It is simply that what may be good for you may be bad for someone else. When you start to build your understanding, you can make those decisions for yourself.

It is important to know what's in your hair care products. Product formulation, or cosmetics chemistry, is a field unto itself. Hundreds of books and thousands of articles have been written on every aspect of it. I am not a professional cosmetics chemist and do not pretend to be one. But I am not an average consumer, either. When it comes to hair care products, I am a pro-consumer—a professional consumer. I consider myself more educated than the average consumer, but not so educated that I am a bona fide scientist or hair care professional.

I am going to provide you with a base of connected information. This information creates a process that can get you started on your way to becoming a professional consumer of hair care products.

I warn you that the reading is not light. I have tried to simplify the information where possible without compromising its correctness. My hope is that you will find the contents of this book understandable and interesting. No subject is so difficult that you can't understand it. Sometimes, the problem may be that whoever is explaining the subject is not doing it in a way you can understand. The failure is not on you, it is on the person providing the information. In this case, that would be me!

This does not excuse you, though. Your job is to find the books, people or information that will help you understand whatever you want to know. Never let an inept or incompetent teacher stop you from learning. I am going to try my best to explain this subject in a way that most of you will understand. I hope I don't get a big fat "fail"! Even if I do not succeed entirely, I hope I can shed light on a few points that will help you.

If you are clear that you want to find a method to help you understand and select hair care products, then please take a deep breath and turn to the next page. You are ready to delve into your hair journey.

CHAPTER 2

Why I Wrote This Book

Dear Ms. Chicoro,
    I have seen this conditioner advertised. The reviews on it are really good, too. Many people are saying how great it works. It sounds like it is really good but ... it's so expensive. The cost is almost $150, but I am thinking of buying it. Here is the name of the product. Could you tell me what you think, please?

The first thing I asked the reader who sent me this email was the list of product ingredients on the back of the label. Never buy a product without looking at the product ingredients first. Here are some ingredients you may find:

- *Sea Water*
- *Cationic Derivatives*
- *Silicone Derivatives*

This list of ingredients is written in a scientific, technical way. The wording is designed to dazzle and confuse you, not to help you understand them. I can tell you that every ingredient listed above, except for the sea water, can be found in inexpensive conditioners you can buy from your local drug store or grocery store for five dollars or even less.

Remember that I have gathered this information after lots and lots of practice and familiarity with the subject. Please don't be intimidated. One's first exposure to any subject is always the hardest. Stay with me! In the end, I think you will be pleasantly surprised by how much you have learned and are able to apply in your own product search.

I have no issues with this product. It might be fun to try it. I did not try to dissuade the lady who sent the email from buying the product. My point is simply that if you are going to buy any product, know what you are getting. Spend your money wisely.

Spending wisely is not defined by what I think or by a certain price point. To spend wisely is to know exactly what you are buying. Know what you want to accomplish, and be clear about how you believe a product will help you reach your hair goals. To purchase a hair product without knowing what the ingredients are, just because they look scientific or magical, is to be a fool with your money. Consumers are dazzled by fancy packaging and words that describe extraordinary benefits and too-good-to-be-true promises. Smoke and mirrors belong on the magician's stage, not in your hair products.

Except for the seawater, all the ingredients from this $150 conditioner can be found in a 79-cent bottle of conditioner from your local store.

You might not mind paying $150 for seaweed-infused water mixed with two or three ingredients that can be found in every home. This product might just solve your most pressing hair issue. But if you are desperate and you believe that a high-cost product will magically change your chewed up, broken off, unhealthy hair into something beautiful, then you are purchasing the product for the wrong reasons.

Billions of dollars are at stake. Cosmetics companies and hair product formulators are now making their ingredient descriptions more scientific and harder for the consumer to understand. This is not because they think you are stupid, but because they know you are smart. You are becoming more sophisticated and more knowledgeable. Their goal is not to fool you, but to entice you to buy. This means you have to step up your game and continue to educate yourself. Do not be distracted. You can learn how to read product labels and understand them without having a degree or certificate in cosmetics chemistry.

New chemicals are synthesized every day, but cosmetics formulation has not changed much in the last hundred years. The names of the ingredients will continue to change, but they fall into categories that are finite and limited.

Product formulation is based on a pattern. When you know the pattern, you can recognize it over and over again. The $150 product follows a pattern. Like most other shampoos and conditioners it is made up of three components:

1. Solvents –This is the liquid base of the product.
2. Surfactant, or a system of surfactants – These are the ingredients in the product that clean, condition and make suds in the product.
3. Additives – These include but are not limited to fragrance, color, vitamins, oils and preservatives in the product.

That's it! This pattern is repeated in every shampoo and conditioner product you buy.

CHAPTER 3

Learn to Decode and Decide for Yourself

The email about the $150 product contains one of the questions I receive most frequently: How do you choose products? I am also asked which products I recommend and what ingredients to look for. The short answer is that it depends on you.

I try to use as few commercially available, on-the-shelf products as possible. I prefer using mainly natural ingredients or products with the smallest possible amount of processing. Well, that's me. It would be naïve to believe that everyone thinks like me. Not everyone has the time or interest or resources to create their own products.

Furthermore, every ingredient or product does not work for every head of hair. Some of the inconsistencies in the results that products provide come from the current state or health of one's hair, any sensitivities or allergies one may have, and personal preferences that have been established through one's culture and lifestyle. The products you select should be based on your knowledge of hair in general, your knowledge of your own unique hair needs and goals, and your knowledge of products and what they are formulated to do. You have to learn all this. You have to work to gain this information. Once you get it, you will have it forever. Then, to stay current, you will need to continue to add to and build upon your knowledge. That's the easy part.

Too often, women want someone to tell them what to buy for their hair and to guarantee that it will provide the results they seek. This does not happen with your relationships, your education, your job or your finances. Why should it happen with your hair care?

There is no such thing as a magical product that is going to solve all your hair problems and help you instantly get the hair of your dreams. But it is possible to solve many of your hair challenges, assuming that you have no health issues that stop you from doing so. It is possible to have healthy, beautiful hair—but you have to be an active part of the process.

If no one can select your hair products for you, then why did I write this book, right? It is because I can provide you with a methodology based on understanding. This methodology is a model or a process that you can use as a framework to determine which ingredients and products are best for you. It will serve as a guide, a systematic approach that you can refine and improve over time.

Putting Afro Hair in Perspective as a Rare, Valuable Commodity

Most studies on hair are conducted using Caucasian and Asian hair. It is difficult for hair research centers to obtain long, unaltered, unprocessed Afro-textured hair. Thus, Afro-textured hair is often simulated for commercial use as wigs.

The practice of the hair care industry is to use Asian hair to represent Afro-textured hair. The Asian hair is treated with alkali, or it is steamed and heat damaged until it crinkles so that it looks "kinky" and curly. There is a difference between hair that is made to look kinky and hair that is naturally kinky. From the very beginning, the hair used and identified as Afro-textured hair that is used for research within the industry and for wigs and extensions is not really Afro-textured hair; it is damaged Asian hair.

You all know those dry, dingy, crunchy, thirsty-looking Afro puffs you see in beauty supply stores. I am pretty sure they didn't come from the head of a person of African descent. I have an aversion to those wigs and hairpieces, but this certainly does not mean that I have an aversion to real, natural Afro-textured hair. Just because somebody calls hair Afro-textured doesn't mean that it is. I think some of those wigs are ugly—not because they are Afro-textured, but because I see them for what they are: fake hair, or natural Asian hair that is made to simulate Afro-textured hair but fails to look like and capture the beauty of natural Afro-textured hair.

Alkali and steam forever break the bonds in your hair that are intended to stay permanently connected. These permanent bonds are called disulfide bonds. They are located in keratin, which makes up the protein in your hair. The steam and steam machines you use at home are okay, because in order to do permanent damage you need high, sustained levels of heat and steam. Most home steamers do not have the capacity to damage your hair in this way.

There are two points to note here. The first point is that when you grow your Afro-textured hair long and do not alter it with chemicals such as those used in relaxing or coloring, your hair has great value from both a cultural and a monetary perspective. It is hard to find this kind of hair in bulk. What's uncommon is valuable. For many people, a person with real, long Afro-textured hair is almost unbelievable. A woman who has taken the time to grow her Afro-textured hair long is an anomaly within some communities. It is unlikely that such a woman will cut her hair and sell it for research. She worked hard to get it. Her hair is invaluable. From a purely economical standpoint, too, long, unaltered Afro-textured hair is very valuable. Don't sell it cheaply. If you are approached about selling your hair for research, understand the value of what you have and negotiate accordingly. Don't laugh! I know of people with Afro-textured hair who have been approached in this way and have sold their hair for research. It does happen. Always try to know and understand your value.

The second point is that simulation is not reality. The great majority of hair that is used for the study of Afro-textured hair is Asian hair, which is a different type. This simulated Afro-textured hair is damaged, but the natural hair that grows from your scalp is not damaged.

My purpose in sharing this information with you is to empower you. I don't want you to perceive the cosmetics industry as an enemy that is paying attention to you now only because they want your money. Look at the industry for what it is. It is in existence to make a profit, and it is at your disposal. You can pick and choose what you want from within the industry. These businesses want your money, so they are responsive to your needs. Your preferences and choices can and do impact the industry.

Are you starting to see the power you wield? Remember, a fool is soon parted from his or her money. In our case, being a fool means being ignorant. Ignorance can be eradicated by knowledge. It's time for you to solidify your knowledge by learning the Four-Step Process.

CHAPTER 4

Overview of the
Hair Products 101 Process

You need only four simple steps to get on the path of being able to choose the right products for yourself. However, simple does not mean easy. Although these steps are simple, they are not easy to implement. Familiarity and practice are essential if you are to master these four steps—or any other skill.

The Four Steps:

1. Understand the human hair fiber
2. Understand your own hair
3. Understand product formulation
4. Put it all together

Step 1: Understanding the Human Hair Fiber

You need to understand the morphological and histological aspects of human hair. Morphology relates to physical characteristics, or the aspects you can see and feel. Histology relates to chemical characteristics. Usually, you cannot see or touch characteristics related to histology.

Step 2: Understanding Your Own Hair

Some of your hair goals may be achievable, and some may not. Examine your hair and document what you see and feel. To assess your hair objectively, you must get your ideas out of your head and put them on paper. This will allow you to look at them from a logical perspective. The key to this step is to learn about your hair, embrace it and accept it. What you should not do is compare your hair to someone else's, or try to make it do something it is just not meant to do.

Step 3: Understanding Product Ingredients and Formulations

In general, store-bought hair products are formulated with specific ingredients for specific reasons. It is important to understand what is in the bottle. It is important to know why a particular ingredient is present and what its purpose is within the overall formulation of the product. Once you understand this, you will find many clues that can help you determine whether the product is for you.

Step 4: Putting It All Together

Step 4 calls you to action. It requires that you do something. It's the step where you need to take action. This step requires you to combine everything you have learned. Now you can use your knowledge to select what's best for you, based on what you have learned from reading this book.

Don't expect it all to make sense immediately. Libraries of books have been written about each of these steps. I know that you are smart, but you are not superhuman. Don't forget that familiarity and practice, time and effort are required to master anything.

CHAPTER 5

Step 1: Understanding the Human Hair Fiber

Physical and Chemical Properties of Healthy Hair

Many books, articles and resources address the structure of the hair fiber. Therefore, I will not go into great detail regarding the science of hair. I will just highlight the important points that relate to hair care products. The most important point is that in general, hair grows approximately ½ inch per month. If your hair seems to stay the same length, then it is most likely breaking as fast as it grows.

Morphological (Physical) Properties

Cuticle

The cuticle consists of scales that overlap. They cover the entire hair strand. In The outermost layer of the hair is the cuticle. The cuticle is the hair strand's first line of defense. To preserve the health of your hair, it is essential to maintain the structure of the cuticle. As you groom your hair, your job is to try to avoid or minimize damage to the cuticle.

Cuticles that are damaged, permanently lifted or missing can create fissures or cracks on the outside of the hair strand. These cracks can penetrate to the cortex of the strand.

Cortex

The cortex is the inner layer of the hair strand and is covered and protected by the cuticle. The cuticle is on the outside and the cortex is on the inside of the hair strand. When the cortex is damaged or degraded, the hair splits and then breaks from the inside out.

Although Afro-textured hair is made up of the same amino acids and proteins as Asian and European hair, Afro hair is unique in many ways. Afro-textured hair strands tend to be more flat than rounded. This means that it does not reflect light the way the other two types of hair do. Afro-textured hair has a beautiful sheen rather than a shine. Also, Afro-textured hair is shaped like a piece of twisted licorice. If you bite off the tip or end a piece of licorice, then peer into the opening, the shape you see is like the shape of afro-textured hair (see figure A). This twisted oval shape of the hair is similar to the shape of licorice.

If you take a strand of Afro-textured hair and elongate it or pull it straight, you will notice that the strand has the shape of a series of footballs connected by sections of straight lines. The footballs, or the rounded parts of the strand, are usually covered by six to eight layers of cuticles. The straighter sections are covered by only two to three layers of cuticles, which means that the straight parts of the hair strand are thinner than the rounded sections. Thus, the straight areas of the strand are more prone to breakage. Also, at the points where the hair strand goes from a curly edge to a straight edge, there may be microscopic, naturally occurring breaks in the hair. This pattern is found in all wavy hair but is more pronounced in Afro-textured hair.

Follicle

The hair follicle is an organelle of the skin. It is a hollow area from which the hair strand grows. The shape of the follicle impacts the shape of the hair strand that grows from within the follicle. Only one hair grows from a follicle at a time.

The Hair Chart by Archetype

Description	African Hair Type	Asian Hair Type	European Hair Type
Shape of strand in cross-section	Elliptical (licorice-shaped)	Circular (tube-shaped)	Oval (egg-shaped)
Shape of strand along its length	Flat, twisted (twists have random reversals in direction along the length of the strand, with possible cracks at the juncture of the twists.)	Rounded, cylindrical	Rounded, ovoid
When combing is easiest	When the hair is wet	When the hair is dry	When the hair is dry
Curve on hair strand	Curved	No curve	Some curve
Shape of inner follicle	Curved	Straight	Slanted
Water absorption	Absorbs the most water, absorbs fastest	Absorbs the least water, absorbs slowly	Absorbs a medium amount of water at a medium rate
Layers of cuticles	6-8 layers on thickest part of strand, 2-3 layers on thinnest part of strand	6-8 layers	6-8 layers
Tensile strength	Not strong	Very strong	Strong
Color	Black, brown	Black	Blonde to black
Breakage	Prone to breakage	Not very prone to breakage	Moderately prone to breakage

Description	African Hair Type	Asian Hair Type	European Hair Type
Average number of hairs on head	50,000 to 100,000 hairs	80,000 to 140,000	86,000 to 146,000 hairs
Grouping of follicles	Follicles usually in groups of three	Follicles in groups of two	Follicles in groups of two
Texture	Curly, kinky	Straight	Straight, wavy or curly
Water Content	Low	High	Medium
Breakage time	Early (not resistant to stress)	Late (resistant to stress)	Medium (moderately resistant to stress)

Archetypes of Hair: Hair Strand Shapes

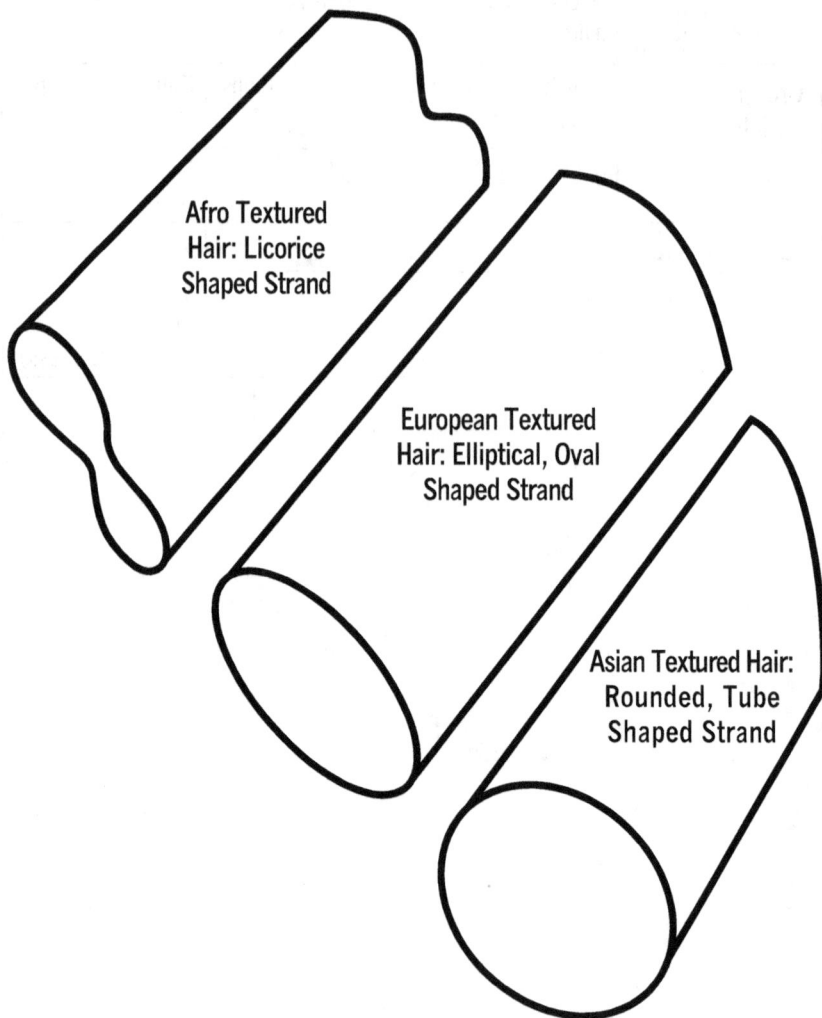

Afro Textured
Hair: Licorice
Shaped Strand

European Textured
Hair: Elliptical, Oval
Shaped Strand

Asian Textured Hair:
Rounded, Tube
Shaped Strand

Figure A

Water or Moisture

Water, or moisture, is one of the most important components of the hair strand. Water maintains the pliability of hair. This means that it makes the hair flexible and bendable.

In order to maintain the highest level of water content in your hair, it is important to air-dry your hair instead of drying it with heating appliances. Hair that is dried naturally will tend to equilibrate with the environment, which means the water content in naturally dried hair will be equal to the water content in the air around you. You want this to happen! Of course, in arid or dry places, such as desert towns, the dry air will dry out your hair. In those cases, it is best to keep your hair moistened and protected or covered.

This is important because Afro-textured hair tends to absorb water faster than other hair textures, but it is not able to absorb as great a total amount of water as other types of hair can. Therefore, Afro-textured hair has to be constantly infused with moisture to keep it pliable, flexible and soft.

When heat from a blow dryer is used, it increases the dryness of your Afro-textured hair. Heat-drying not only removes the excess water that makes the hair wet, it dries the hair beyond the point where its natural moisture levels need to be. Hair that has been heat-dried cannot equilibrate to, or match, the moisture level in the air around it. To make the moisture level in the hair equal to the moisture level in the air, you will have to re-saturate your hair and then let it dry naturally. Heat-drying the hair brings it to a state of unnatural dryness, and constant dryness hastens damage to the hair strand.

Without water, the hair shaft or strand can fracture and break. None of us can control the air in the environment, but you can manage your hair's moisture level by creating an environment for your hair. Do this by fixing a plastic sandwich bag on your ponytail or a plastic shower cap over your entire head. These are methods of protective styling. Many people in the home hair care world refer to these methods as the "baggie method" and the "whole head baggie method." These methods keep the hair moist.

Remember, it's water that keeps hair moist, not oil or grease. Oil and grease provide lubrication to the hair, but only water gives a real change in the moisture content of the hair strand. Moisture is water. Lubrication is oil. Aloe vera can be used to moisturize hair, too, since much of the content of aloe vera is water. Glycerin and silicone make hair feel softer and moister, but this is a tactile change, or a change in the way the hair feels. It is not a real change in the moisture content.

Electric Conductivity

Electric conductivity is another physical property of hair. Two types of electrical charges may impact the hair. One is called triboelectricity, and the other is called piezoelectricity. Triboelectricity is an electric charge that comes from friction, such as when hair rubs against cloth. Piezoelectricity is an electric charge that comes from pressure, such as when a comb is run through or against the hair.

Natural Afro-textured hair, which has some curl, rarely exhibits flyaway hair. If you heat-straighten your hair, you increase your chances of experiencing static electricity, or flyaway hair.

Physical Bonds

Hair is made up proteins and elements that are linked by three kinds of bonds. Two of the bonds are physical and one of the bonds is chemical. The two physical bonds are salt bonds and hydrogen bonds. Both are temporary and are easy to form and break. They are water-dependent.

When you wet your hair, the water inserts itself between the salt or hydrogen bonds, breaking them. When you dry your hair, the salt bonds re-form and take whatever shape the hairs were arranged in when it was wet. This is what leaves curls after a wet set has dried.

If heat is applied to the hair, it breaks the salt bonds and leaves the hair straight. That is why the heat of warm water relaxes curls and makes Afro-textured hair easier to detangle. Heating implements such as ceramic flat irons straighten the hair by heating it from the inside to the outside. Non-ceramic flat irons straighten the hair by heating it from the outside in. Ceramic flat irons may be better for the hair because they straighten it more quickly than the non-ceramic kind, thus removing less moisture from the hair. A non-ceramic flat iron can take longer to straighten the hair, allowing for more moisture to be lost.

Histological (Chemical) Properties

Disulfide (Disulphide) Bonds

Disulfide bonds are chemical bonds. They contain sulfur. Unlike the physical bonds of salt and hydrogen, once the disulfide bonds are broken they do not re-form or return to their original, natural state. These bonds are broken and re-formed by relaxers and permanent wave procedures, and they are completely dissolved by the ingredients in hair removers.

Charge

Products and cosmetics for the hair use charges to bind to the hair. To learn how to select products, it is essential that you have an understanding of the relation between the charges in the product ingredients and the charge on the hair.

There are four types of charges found in substances:

1. (-) anionic—negative charge.
2. (0) nonionic—no charge.
3. (+) cationic—positive charge.
4. (-/+) zwitterionic – positive and negative charge.

Anionic	Nonionic	Cationic	Zwitterionic
(-) Negatively Charged	(0) Neutrally Charged	(+) Positively Charged	(+ and -) Positively and Negatively Charged

The majority of the interaction between the hair strand and external forces takes place on the surface of the cuticle, so it is the cuticle, or the surface of the hair, that becomes charged. Therefore, most hair care products are formulated to act upon the cuticle. pH is the measure of how acid or how basic is the solution. The scale used is based on 14. From 0 to 6 is considered acidic, 7 is considered neutral and 8 to 12 is considered basic. Since water has a pH of 7.0, most products are formulated with the assumption that hair has a negative charge.

You already know that water is a vital component of hair. Hair is hygroscopic, which means that it naturally attracts water.

Physical and Chemical Properties of Damaged Hair

Tangles

Believe or not, the most damage is done to hair by other hair on the same head! The rubbing of hair on hair does more damage than the rubbing of mechanical implements such as brushes or combs. This is one reason you should try to avoid getting tangles in your precious hair.

If you take one strand of hair and hold it between two fingers, you are holding the diameter, or the diametrical view, of the hair. If you stretch the hair and hold the end in one hand and the part near the root in the other hand, you are looking at the longitudinal, or lengthwise, view of the hair. The worst kind of damage is done to your hair when you remove or comb out tangles. When you comb or brush through a tangle, significant pressure is applied to the hair, especially at the point where you snatch or pull through the tangle. In addition to this, the hair is being bent as you try to brush the tangle out. This pressure and bending impacts the diameter of the hair, and a split may begin to form at this point. Once the hair splits, it is permanently damaged and can never be repaired. If you want healthy, longer hair, you need to avoid splits. That is why you should try to avoid tangles. If you can't avoid them, try to detangle your hair as gently as possible.

Weathering

The disulfide bonds of the hair contain cystine, an amino acid rich in sulfur. When exposed to sun, wind and bleaching, the cystine is oxidized, or turned into cysteic acid. Cysteic acid is not a natural component of human hair. It comes from the breakdown or degradation of the cystine amino acid in the hair, which is caused by exposure to sun, wind and the environment and from bleaching the hair. If the weathering is natural, the cysteic acid will be concentrated on the ends of the hair. If the damage is caused by bleaching, the cysteic acid will most likely be distributed along the entire strand, wherever it was bleached. In both cases, the hair has been chemically damaged.

Virgin or unprocessed hair tends to by hydrophobic, which means that it dislikes or repels water. In contrast, chemically damaged hair is hydrophilic, which means that it is attracted to water. It is also more negatively charged, which makes it dry. Hair that is chemically damaged from bleaching and coloring and from the environment is thirsty! Damaged hair is porous; it can't keep water in (or out) as well as non-damaged hair can.

The more natural your hair is, the less chemically damaged it will be and the less product you will need to use. This doesn't mean that healthy Afro-textured hair can get away with only a dime-sized amount of product, but you need less product on healthy Afro-textured hair than on unhealthy or damaged hair.

As already mentioned, healthy hair tends to be hydrophobic. In other words, healthy hair doesn't like water to penetrate it. People with Afro-textured hair often complain that water just sits on top of their hair. That's a good thing. It means the hair is healthy and is doing its job: repelling water.

Signs of Damaged Hair

Tangles   The hair may have too much friction, or particles of frayed hair may be catching on other hairs.

Lifted cuticles   The hair strand feels rough.

Oxidization   The hair is discolored or the ends feel sticky.

Fracture Patterns

Repetitive actions such as washing, detangling and styling can damage your hair. The average consumer recognizes this damage as split ends and broken hair. Splitting is only one of the ways that the hair can break or fracture.

Hair can break in five different fracture patterns. The five fracture patterns are step, fibrillated, split-ended, smooth and angled. Afro-textured hair tends to experience predominantly three of the five fracture patterns: step fracture, fibrillated fracture and the split end fracture.

Step Fracture

The step fracture is the most common fracture pattern in Afro-textured hair. The step fracture occurs along the diameter of the hair strand. This fracture is related to the water content in the hair. Remember, Afro-textured hair absorbs water faster than other hair types, but it is able to absorb a smaller total amount than the other types. When the hair swells with water, it gets "fatter," which means that it swells diametrically; at the same time, it stretches, or gets longer. The resulting tension in the strand causes breakage. This is the most common way that Afro-textured hair breaks.

Fibrillated Fracture

The fibrillated fracture is the second most common pattern of breakage in Afro-textured hair. The fibrillated fracture is not a smooth or clean break. Think of a fabric that has dry rot. It is dry and fragile and almost breaks apart, and the ends of the fabric are often fuzzy or frayed. Fibrillated fractures occur when the inner part of the hair strand becomes misaligned and unstable. This causes the hair to fray.

Split-Ended Fracture

The split-ended fracture is the third most common breaking pattern in Afro-textured hair. Most people are familiar with this type of break. Hair can split at any point on the hair shaft, but when the break occurs most noticeably on the end of the hair, it is called a split-ended fracture.

Smooth Fracture

Smooth fractures occur most often on non-Afro-textured hair. These fractures are clean breaks of the hair strand. They are likely to occur when wet hair is brushed or combed. This is why you often hear people say you should never brush or comb wet hair.

However, since smooth fractures occur most often in wavy Caucasian hair, it is Caucasian hair that should not be brushed wet or combed when wet. In the case of Afro-textured hair, water relaxes the curl on the hair strand. Thus, when using a tool such as comb or brush, it is better to detangle Afro-textured hair when it is wet. Neither Caucasian nor Afro-textured hair should be combed too aggressively.

In general, I advocate finger-combing or detangling Afro-textured hair when it is dry, but under specific conditions. First the hair should be free of product. It should not be gummy, sticky or hardened with product. Second, use only your fingers. Third, the goal is not to get the hair tangle-free all at once, but to section the hair so that you can work on small areas, one at a time.

If all these conditions cannot be met, then Afro-textured hair is to be detangled with a comb when the hair is wet. Only if the hair is tangle-free and product-free should it be combed through when dry.

Basically, the curlier your natural hair is, the more likely it is that you should detangle it wet. The straighter your natural hair is, the less likely it is that you should detangle it wet. You have to decide in which category your hair falls.

Angled Fracture

The last kind of fracture is the angled fracture. Angled fractures are breaks that occur at an angle on the hair strand. These types of fractures are not commonly experienced on Afro-textured hair.

Hair Fracture Patterns

Step

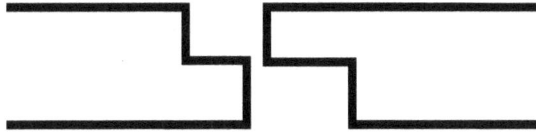

Fibrillated

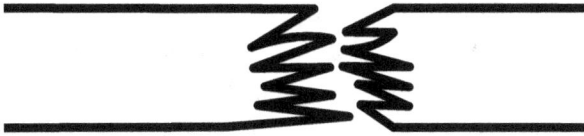

Split Ended

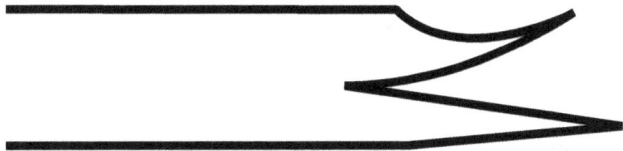

Smooth

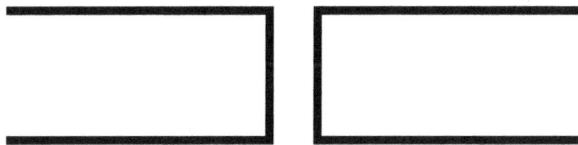

Angled

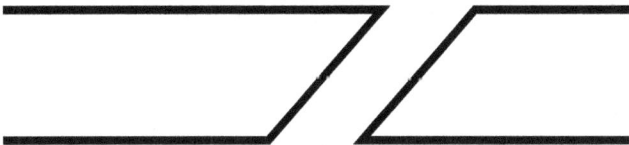

(Kalmath, 1984)

Forces that Act on the Hair

A force is any influence on a substance, body, or system that produces a change in its movement or shape. The two main forces that impact the hair are friction and gravity.

Friction

The most important force on the hair is friction. Friction means rubbing. Frictional characteristics concern the way hair interacts with other hair. Hair that has low frictional characteristics is hair that is healthy or not very damaged. Healthy hair should naturally move and align in the same direction as the bulk of the hair on the head. Slippage means that the hairs easily move over one another; they don't feel sticky or gummy. Product-free, natural hair should have natural slippage.

If hair is sticky when it has no product on it, it has likely been damaged. The more damaged your hair is, the more friction and the less slip it will have. That is why consistently tangled hair may be damaged hair. Conditioning agents such as oil and silicone provide lubrication, or slippage, so that hairs can move easily over one another.

Healthy hair has something called a directional frictional effect (DFE). This is what allows hairs to move easily across one another and align themselves in the same direction. When your hair is damaged, it loses this DFE.

Basically, the cuticles of the hair lie along the strand in the same direction, from the root to the tip. If you rub your hair from the root to the tip, you are moving in the direction of the way the cuticles lie on a healthy strand. If you rub your hair from tip to root, you are rubbing against the grain, or against the direction of the cuticle. This creates friction. The more friction hair has, the less DFE it has.

Gravity

Gravity is the other important force that relates to hair. Tensile strength is defined as how prone your hair is to breakage. In other words, tensile strength is the ability of the hair to stand up to gravity. Healthy hair has excellent tensile strength.

Think of a weight tied to the end of a string. The string represents the hair, and the weight could represent a heavy ponytail holder. The tensile strength of the string is demonstrated by how well it can withstand the heaviness of the weight without breaking.

Many girls wear barrettes, beads or weighted objects on the ends of their ponytails. These weighted objects exert a gravitational force on the hair. Tensile strength determines at which point the hair breaks because of the weight pulling down on it. In general, if you want to preserve your hair, it is best not to place weighted objects on the ends of your hair.

Additional Forces

Other forces that act on the hair are torsion and compression.

Torsion means the state of being twisted. The hair strands of Afro-textured hair twist naturally. The strand may be flat, but it twists like a piece of licorice. Because of this natural twist, a single strand can reverse its direction many times. This is one reason Afro-textured hair has a tendency to knot. This kind of knot is often referred to as a single-strand knot.

Because of the twisting or curvature on the hair strand, the cuticles on healthy Afro-textured hair tend to lift naturally and stay more lifted than the cuticles on straighter hair. This leads to a tendency to have microscopic tears in areas of the strand where the hair changes direction. These tears are not due to damage but to the frequent changes in direction of the naturally twisted strand. If you have ever watched a documentary on reptiles and seen a snake turn and twist, you have seen its scales lift at the points where its body curves. That will give you an idea of what the lifted cuticles look like on a natural curl of Afro-textured hair.

Compression is the pressing, squeezing or holding of your hair strands. Compression is important because you can apply it to your hair when you are trying to detangle it. You can twist or squeeze and hold the hair above a tangle to release some of the pressure on the hair below the tangle, where you are trying to comb it through. This may help to minimize over-stretching the hair and cut down on breakage during detangling.

Much more information has been written about hair, but further details are not necessary here. We've reviewed the basic structure and nature of hair in general. The next step is to take some time with your own hair. Understanding your hair is step two in the process.

CHAPTER 6

Step 2: Understanding Your Own Hair

This is the easiest step in the entire process, because you don't need any external information to perform it. However, if you are not accustomed to being honest and fair with yourself, it can also be the most difficult step.

Write It Down

Before you start to answer the questions in this chapter, flip through the book until you find the template at the end of the chapter. You can use it to record your answers. You might even want to make a few copies of it. Or you may want to skip it altogether and write your answers directly in a notebook of your own.

If you are critical—if you always find something wrong with yourself—you are not being fair to yourself. Far too many of us live our lives this way. As you read this book, try to suspend such criticism. There are no correct or incorrect answers here. What you are doing is gathering information about your hair. The more you know about your hair, the better decisions you can make.

Be honest with yourself. Make a fair assessment about the state of your hair and how you feel about it. No one else has to know what you think or feel. You only have to document what you see and know about your hair. Write it down.

Keeping a written record is as essential as keeping a photographic record of your hair. When you make notes, make sure you are doing it in such a way that later on you will be able to pick up your notebook and understand what you have written. It is a waste of time to scribble ugly, illegible notes that you won't be able to read after today. Take your time and write it right! Be thorough and meticulous. You want to have to do this only one time, and then refine it. You don't want to have to go back and re-do the whole thing because your initial work was sloppy.

Photograph and Document Your Hair

If you have not already done so, I would strongly suggest that you take photographs of your hair as soon as possible. Take at least six photographs: one of the left side of your hair, one of the right side, one of the top of your head, one of the back, and one each of the front right and left edges of your hairline.

These photos are your record of where you are today. Some people ask me if they should wait until they have started to see improvement. But if you have nothing to compare the future photos with, how are you going to know if you are seeing any improvement? You won't.

Take the pictures now. They will serve as the baseline or starting point for your journey. Print the photos, label and date them, and place them in a notebook or post them online where you can see them. This is an important step. Progress that our eyes do not detect can be recorded in photographs. Remember, you are not required to show these photographs to anyone. You are the only one who needs to see them.

Identify and Document the Condition of Your Scalp and Hair

Examine your scalp and hair without being overly critical. Try to be as objective and factual as you can without focusing on your hair in a purely negative or emotional way. This is easier said than done, but you can do it.

The categories you are going to document are how your hair looks, feels, moves and smells. You did not read that incorrectly. I did say smells! Write down whether or not your hair is natural, texlaxed, transitioning, permanently waved, bleached and/or colored. This information will help you be clear when it comes to selecting the product that will provide the results you want.

Your Scalp

How Does Your Scalp Look?

Your hair follicles are deep within your scalp. Unlike your hair, which is made of dead, hardened protein, your scalp is made of skin that is alive. It usually will be much lighter than the skin on your face and body.

First look at you scalp to see if it is coated. In general, you should avoid scratching your scalp with your nail or any kind of implement, but now is the exception. Go ahead. Lightly and gently scratch the surface of a tiny area with your fingernail. If you see any scales or skin on your nails and fingers, you may have some scalp issues. If your scalp is painful to the touch, if you have any open wounds or sores, or if you have severe flaking, please go and see a dermatologist. Remember, you need to focus on yourself. You need to take care of yourself.

How Does Your Scalp Feel?

You have already touched your scalp. Does it feel dry and crusty? Does it feel soft and smooth? Even if you determine that a visit to the doctor is in order, you still need to know what is going on with your own body. You know your body better than anyone. The more you know about yourself, the sooner you can detect if there is something that is not working the way it should be. Your doctor is not responsible for the early detection of issues in or on your body, you are. Write down the information.

How Does Your Scalp Smell?

Now that you have touched your scalp, sniff your fingers. This may seem weird, but smells are important. They are indicators of disease, poison, illness and internal imbalances. If there is an odor, note it in your documentation. If there is not an odor, document that as well. Now let's move on to your hair.

Your Hair

How Does Your Hair Look?

State

What is the state of your hair? Is it relaxed, natural, transitioning, permanently waved, bleached, colored and/or tex-laxed? Write this information down and keep it in your documentation.

Transitioning hair is the most complex hair to manage. That is because when you are transitioning, you have two distinct textures of hair on your head: natural and chemically processed. The two textures may respond differently to the same products.

Style

How do you wear your hair? Do you wear it loose or do you employ protective styling? Do you use heat to style your hair? If so, how often? What kind of heat do you use? What types of materials do you use in your hair: nylon, cotton, silk, satin, metal? Think about this and write your answers.

Shine or Sheen

Afro-textured hair may not look shiny without some type of lubrication, because the strand of Afro-textured hair is flattened rather than rounded or cylindrical. Instead of shine, your hair may have a beautiful sheen. A sheen on the hair may not be as brilliant as a shine, but it can be just as pretty.

If your hair is dull or coated-looking, please note that as well. Hair that has been weathered or damaged may have tips or ends that are whitened or gray. This is easier to see on heat-straightened hair, but natural hair is not immune to this type of damage.

Color

Is your hair color-treated, dyed or bleached? Hair in this category tends to be more porous and thirsty. It is important to note this detail if it applies to your hair.

Texture

What is the texture of your hair? Does your hair look roughened to your own eyes? Is it fuzzy-looking? Do you think it is puffy? Does it look thin or thick?

If you have had your hair cut in layers, jot down this information here. Hair that has been cut in layers can appear fuzzy or frizzy because of the different lengths. This does not mean it's unhealthy. With layered hair, you are seeing mostly the ends or tips of the hair at every layer instead of seeing the middle part of the strands. This may give the overall head of hair a fuzzy, dull, weathered look. Make sure you are aware of this. If you have layered hair, look at the actual strands of hair and not just the ends.

Strands

Examine the individual hair strands within your hair. Are they split or frayed in the middle? Are they thin, thick or average-looking to you? Do they look different from how you remember them in the past? Write down whatever comes to mind as you gaze at your hair strands. Remember, there is no wrong or right information. Learn to trust yourself.

Ends

Take a look at the tips or ends of your hair. Are they thinner than the rest of the hair on your head? Is there any crunchiness or dryness on your hair ends? Are they lighter in color than the rest of your hair? Do you see lots of split ends or little knots near the ends of your hair? Are the ends even or scraggly? Have the ends of your hair been recently trimmed or cut, or has it been a while since you had a trim? Write down what you observe, and add any dates that indicate when you last had your hair trimmed or cut. If you don't remember, that's okay. Please don't fuss at yourself or berate yourself.

What Do You Like?

Take a moment to look back over the notes you have made thus far. What are your thoughts and feelings about your hair overall? Do you want to remove it as if it were a wig and pass it on to someone to take care of it for you? Unless your hair is not real, that's not going to happen!

How do you feel about your hair? Are you overwhelmed and confused? Do you like your hair? Do you wish you had hair like someone else's? Have you ever liked your own natural hair? Has anyone ever complimented you on how pretty your hair was? Has anyone ever made a negative comment about your hair? Write down what feels safe and what feels scary. The more you know about how you feel about your hair, the sooner you can address what it needs to get it on track with the right treatment and products.

What Don't You Like?

Most of us are so mired in negativity, whether it be from external or internal influences and sources, that this part usually comes the easiest. Since that is the case, I want you to limit yourself to three comments. Pick the top three things that you don't like about your hair and write them down.

What Do You Want Your Hair to Look Like?

Avoid comparing your hair to someone else's. Often, we use comparisons to focus on what is wrong with us or what makes us better than someone else. Let's just focus on your hair.

Think about how your hair was when you were little or at a point in your life when you liked it the most. What was wonderful about it? As memories come to mind, take notes. The hair that you are envisioning is probably the goal for you.

Your hair goal is not where you are right now, but it has to be something that is possible for you. The hair in your past that you liked is a tangible goal for your future. If you can, get a photo of your hair from that time. Make a copy of it and put in your notebook, or wherever you are documenting your hair information.

If you have never liked your hair, ask yourself why. If you are not focused on the health of your hair but on wishing that something about your hair was different, your issue may not be related to product selection. Your challenge may be that you need to learn to accept yourself.

How Does Your Hair Feel?

Roots

How do the roots of your hair feel? I have heard many transitioning women refer to the natural, chemical-free hair that is growing from their scalps as scab hair. This is a term for hair that feels roughened. My understanding is that hair growing from your scalp should feel rougher than freshly relaxed hair. That is because it has all its cuticles intact.

This newly-grown hair is the healthiest hair on the entire head. Feel the strands as close to the roots as you can. How do your roots feel? Now pull away from the root and go down the hair strand to the tip or end of the hair strand. How does it feel from root to tip? It's okay to compare the root to the strand and the strand to the tip. It's your hair. Write down your experience.

Strands

Focus on your strands. Are they bumpy and rough? Does your finger catch on the strand as you move down it? Cuticles lie downward, towards the ends, and the hair strand will feel smoother if you rub down it from the root to the end. Even healthy hair will feel rougher if you rub it upward, from tip to root, because that is against the way the cuticles lie.

Ends

The ends of your hair are the oldest part of the hair strands. How do they feel? Are they wispy and thin? Do they feel much finer or thinner than the rest of your hair? Do they feel drier and more brittle? Are they soft and supple? Document this information.

How Does Your Hair Move?

Now focus on the bulk or majority of your hair. Shake your head and turn it from side to side. What do you notice?

How Does the Bulk of the Hair Move?

Does your hair move at all, or is it caked and gummy with product? Is it stiff, dry and brittle? Does your hair bounce like a rubber ball? Does it hold steady like a ball of cotton? Does it hang limp and lifeless?

Maybe your hair doesn't move. That's okay, too. Some hair is very healthy but it doesn't move. Write down the information. You are collecting data, not judging it.

How Do Individual Sections of the Hair Move?

What about your strands of hair? When you pull and separate a few hairs from the bulk of the hair, do they stand straight out? Or do the hairs seem longer than the rest for a moment and then spring back into place? What happens to your hair when you separate a piece? All this information is important.

Maybe the individual sections of your hair don't move, either. Again, it is not important to judge this as a good thing or a bad thing. Just make a note and add it to what you have already written.

How Does Your Hair Smell?

Document whether or not there is a discernable smell. If there is a smell, describe it. Perhaps your hair is perfumed from the products you are using. Maybe it smells burnt because you used a too-hot heating tool. Maybe it smells like sulfur. Or maybe it just smells bad because you need to wash it. For now, it's all good. We are observing and documenting. Please reserve judgment as best as you can.

Creating a Baseline for You

Whether you want to do all these steps or not is up to you. You may gravitate to some steps and not want to be bothered with others. By answering these questions, you are establishing a baseline of detailed information about the current state of your hair. This will give you something to compare your hair with later on to see if there has been a change, for better or for worse. Not only will you know that there has been a change, you will know exactly what the change is and when it began. That is definitive, accurate, fact-based information. You can work with it.

This is a model, a process. A model is a structure, and in order to function, the structure requires data and input. For a process to function at an optimum level, it has to have good information put into it. Do yourself a favor and put accurate, detailed information into your model or process.

Your Routine

Regimen

People often say they have no hair routine. Just because it is not well thought out or formal does not mean that your hair routine does not exist. It does.

Whatever you are doing to your hair is your routine. If you get it washed every two weeks and only curl it between those days, that's your routine. Write it down. If you have an idea of what you do and when you do it, write it down. If you do a monthly cleansing that is different than your weekly cleansing, be sure to jot that down, as well. Make the distinction clear and identify what is part of your weekly routine and of your monthly routine, or whatever it is that you are doing.

Your Products

This next step requires a considerable amount of effort. I suggest you follow this step for no more than three products, as a start. You must work to gather information, but you don't want the work to be so hard that it makes you quit. If you have little ones in the house, you can make a game of asking them to help you with the colors and smells of the products. If the children are older, maybe they can help you read the little bitty print on the back of the bottles, or at least spell it out for you.

If you are interested in hair, you probably have many products. The products you use the most are considered your staple products. For most people, these staple products will consist of a shampoo, a conditioner and a moisturizing or protein treatment. You might have some type of leave-in product, as well. For each of these products, please write down the following information.

Name

What is the name of the product? Who makes it? Don't just write "shampoo," write the whole title. If the product is called "Funky Goo Cleaner," that's what you should write.

Color of Packaging

Look at the bottle. What colors do you see? I love the color purple. Many of the products I used to buy had purple somewhere on the bottle, or the writing was purple. When products are packaged in purple, I have to be on guard because I have a tendency to gravitate to those products and buy them, whether I need them or not.

Shape of the Container

What about the shape of the bottle? Do you find it cute and attractive? Is the shape sleek and sexy? I like the way some containers are shaped. This doesn't mean I only buy products according to the shape of their containers, but I'll buy a daintily shaped bottle that fits perfectly in my little hand sooner than one in a bulky jar. Do you notice that you buy products whose containers have similar shapes?

Fragrance

How does the product smell? Is it fruity or musky? Is it sweet like food, or sweet like perfume? Is scent not important to you, or is it very important to you? Write down your answer.

Consistency

What about the texture of the product? Is it watery and runny? Is it thick like a paste? Is it smooth and creamy? You might be attracted to the consistency of a product. I like textures that are smooth, thick and creamy.

Color

What color is the product? Is it pastel pink or electric yellow? Does it matter to you? Is it shiny and pearlescent? Does it sparkle or have particles of something in it? Maybe you like products that are white.

Ingredients

What are the first ten ingredients in each of your staple products? For now, just write down the first ten. If a product has fewer than ten ingredients, write all of them. You are not going to analyze them now. You just want to document them.

Purpose

Look at the writing on the front or back of the container. What is the product verbiage? What do the words convey that this product will do for you? What is the promise? Will it make dry, brittle hair soft and moist? Will it tame unmanageable hair? You don't have to write everything down, just the main idea that speaks to you. What words on the bottle resonated with you, got you breathing fast and made your heart pump? Basically, what were the words or phrases on the bottle that made you pick it up and buy it?

How Did the Product Come to Your Attention?

Why did you buy this product? Was it because someone recommended it to you? Did you see it advertised? Did you meet someone with hair you admire and find out that she uses it? Try to think about and remember why you spent your money to obtain this product.

How Often Do You Use It?

How frequently do you use this product? Do you use it daily, weekly, monthly, or every three months?

Where Do You Use It?

Do you use the product on your scalp? Or, do you use it on your roots? Maybe you use this product exclusively on your hair tips. Or maybe you don't know where you are supposed to use it.

What Do You Expect It to Do for Your Hair?

What is this product supposed to do for your hair? Here we're interested not in what the bottle says but in what you thought. Did you want it to make your hair look like the hair of the lady on the bottle? Were you trying to get your hair to look like that of someone you have seen or someone you know? Or were you trying to resolve a specific hair challenge or problem? Maybe you purchased it because you have always bought it, or because it's inexpensive. You know the routine by now: Write it down, please! Try to be honest. It may not feel good now, but that's okay. It's part of the process.

Does the product work for you the way you want it to? If it does, write "yes" and the reason you are satisfied with it. If it does not, write down the reason you are disappointed with the product.

Now, please go back through this product section and answer the same questions for all your staple products.

Your Life

Believe it or not, what is going on in your life can impact your hair. Food, and specifically an insufficient intake of protein, can impact your hair. If you can afford to purchase this book, it is unlikely that you have a lack of protein in your diet or that you are experiencing severe malnutrition from a lack of eating. Therefore, I will not address food as it relates to hair.

I will focus on two kinds of events in life that can affect your hair: time-related events and trauma-related events. Sometimes they are the same.

Time-Related Events

When someone notices an issue that has arisen with her hair in connection with a life event, it usually happens within what I call a two-year-to-two-week window. If you have experienced changes to your hair, think about what life changes you have undergone anywhere between the last two years and the last two weeks.

This may seem ridiculous at first. How can you remember such details? You'll be surprised at what pops up and what you remember. Have you changed or lost a job? Has your job become more stressful? Have you started going back to school? Have you had a child? Have you lost a child or parent, friend or lover? Have you gained weight? Have your finances changed? Try to write down the event and the time period in which it occurred.

All these life events can affect you emotionally, and the emotional effects can manifest physically as adverse changes to your hair. Be conscious of what is going on around you and inside you. Your body, including your hair, is always giving you clues and information about what is going on. Pay attention. That's not your doctor's or beautician's job. It's your job!

Understanding Your Hair: The Template

Part I: This is where you perform an external analysis. This will help you to see what you are doing to your hair and what effects your actions are having.

Photographs

Take photographs of the following six areas and describe what you see.

Left side:

_____

_____

Right side:

_____

_____

Top of head:

_____

_____

Nape (back of the neck):

_____

_____

Right hairline:

_____

_____

Left hairline:

_____

_____

1. Condition of Scalp
    A. My scalp looks …

    _____

    _____

    B. My scalp feels …

    _____

    _____

    C. My scalp smells …

    _____

    _____

2. Condition of Hair
    A. How It Looks
        i. The state of my hair is …

        _____

        _____

        ii. I usually wear my hair styled …

        _____

        _____

        iii. I use heat in the form of …

        _____

        _____

iv. The number of times I use heat per month is ...

_____

_____

v. In my hair, I usually use (nylon/cotton/silk/satin/metal) ...

_____

_____

vi. The sheen on my hair is

_____

_____

vii. I color my hair _____ times per year using:
    a. I use permanent dye. The brand and color are ...

_____

_____

    I use bleach. The brand is ...

_____

_____

    b. I highlight my hair. I use ...

_____

_____

viii. Texture
    a. My hair texture is ...

_____

_____

    b. Other information about my hair texture is ...

_____

_____

c. My hair is layered (where) ...

_____

_____

d. My hair strands are ...
   i. split

_____

_____

   ii. frayed

_____

_____

   iii. knotted

_____

_____

   iv. other observations

_____

_____

ix. My hair tips are ...
  a. split

_____

_____

  b. frayed

_____

_____

  c. weathered (whitish, grayish)

_____

_____

d. knotted

_____

_____

e. other observations

_____

_____

x. What I like about my hair:

_____

_____

_____

_____

_____

_____

xi. What I don't like about my hair:

_____

_____

_____

_____

_____

_____

xii. How my ideal hair looks:

_____

_____

_____

_____

_____

_____

xiii. How my hair looked when I was a child (if possible, get a photo and put it with your other photos):

_____

_____

_____

_____

_____

_____

B. How my hair feels
   i. The roots feel like ...

_____

_____

_____

_____

   ii. The strands feel like ...

_____

_____

_____

_____

   iii. The ends feel like ...

_____

_____

_____

_____

C. How My Hair Moves
   i. The bulk of my hair moves like

_____

_____

_____

ii. The sections or strands of my hair move like …

_____

_____

_____

D. How My Hair Smells
   i. My hair smells like …

_____

_____

_____

ii. I like/dislike how my hair smells because

_____

_____

_____

Baseline

Review the notes you have taken. Try to summarize the condition and state of your hair. Use the information that you documented in this template to help you. Just write down what jumps out at you. You may just copy something you have already written or you may write down a conclusion you have arrived at or an epiphany you have realized.

_____

_____

_____

_____

_____

_____

_____

_____

Summary

Describe and summarize your thoughts about your hair. Just look over the information that you have documented thus far. Jot down whatever comes to mind on the lines below.

_____

_____

_____

_____

_____

_____

_____

_____

Regimen

What is your regimen? Describe how you wash and care for your hair.

_____

_____

_____

_____

_____

_____

What Products Do You Use?
(Select three for now.)

Product name			
Maker of product			
Color of bottle or container			
Shape of container			
Fragrance of product			
Consistency of product			
Color of product			
Product ingredients			
Purpose of product			
How did you find this product?			
How often do you use it?			
Where on your hair do you use it?			
Does it work the way you expected?			

Part II: This is where you perform an internal analysis. This will help you to see or make any emotional connections to what is manifesting with your hair.

Condition of Life

Think about the last two years until today.

A. Have you gotten a new job?

B. Have you lost a job?

C. Has there been a death or a debilitating illness in your family or someone close to you?

D. Have you become ill or debilitated?

E. Have you been placed on medication or had your medicine changed?

F. Have you experienced an upswing in your finances?

G. Have you experienced a downswing in your finances?

H. Have you bought a new house?

I. Have you lost your house?

J. Have you moved out on your own?

K. Have you started school?

L. Have you finished school?

M. Have you begun a relationship?

N. Have you ended a relationship?

O. Has the relationship dramatically changed from what it used to be?

P. Have you had a new baby?

Q. Has something important to you come into your life?

R. Has something important to you left your life?

S. Have you changed your diet significantly?

T. Have you eliminated a food or drink from your diet?

U. Have you added a food or drink?

V. Have you added or eliminated a supplement?

Why Are You Doing This?

As you notice, there is no scoring. There are no suggested explanations, either. By answering these questions as truthfully as you can, you can determine many things about yourself, specifically about your hair and the habits associated with it.

Your habits are neither bad nor good. They are simply your habits. The more you understand about them, the more insights you can gain about yourself. You may start seeing a pattern in how you purchase your hair products. This pattern may help you continue to buy what is working for you, or it may help you become conscious of habits that drive you toward products you should stay away from. They are products that don't work for you.

If something is in a pretty package with purple writing and it smells good, whether it is natural or not it will be in my basket ready to be purchased unless I stop and think. These questions and answers may help to make you aware of what you do so that you can identify your vulnerabilities. Remember, knowledge is power.

All this information may seem like overkill. It's not. Most people spend most of their time thinking about themselves, anyway. Why not use that time to help you get where you want to go?

Most of the thinking that people do about themselves is in the form of worry or fear. If you are going to focus on yourself, this is one way to make it productive. It is not a waste of time. Once you become aware of this information, it will forever be in the back of your mind. Or, if you have followed my suggestion, it will forever be written down in your notebook. The more self-aware you become, the more thoughtful your choices and decisions will be. The better decisions you make for yourself, the better off you and those around you will be.

By now, you should have a general understanding of hair, and you have a sense of the state of your hair and where you want to go with it. You also know what you use and why you are using it, even if it's just because it smells good. It's time to focus on product ingredients. Here we go.

CHAPTER 7

Step 3: Understanding Product Ingredients & Formulations

Overview of Hair Care Products

"Hi. I have collarbone-length hair, but my hair is dry and dull. What product should I use to get rid of my dryness?"

This is an example of the kind of question I frequently receive. It is a good question, but more information is needed before a good answer can be provided.

Whether this person realizes or not, she is looking for a magic product or a magic answer. By now, you know that neither exists. She would like me to tell her what to use to instantly resolve her hair issues. All I know about her is that her hair is dry and that it is at collarbone length. I need more information.

I can easily tell her to increase the moisture in her hair by adding more water to it. In general, that would be correct, but it would not help her. Although her question does not state it, she is looking for a specific answer based upon her specific situation and needs.

Think about what you have learned so far. What questions might you ask this person? First I would ask what products she is using. What are the ingredients? Then I would ask about her routine and the state of her hair. I usually ask people first about their products and ingredients, because these questions are easy for them to answer. Later I ask about the state of their hair and their hair goals. These questions require more thought. My goal is to help and empower people, not intimidate them or make them feel bad.

We've talked about hair and goals. Now it's time to focus on product ingredients and formulations.

Ionic Bonding

The formulation of hair care products is based upon the chemistry of ionic bonding, or the relationship between negative and positive charges. In order to be able to select the best shampoo and conditioner for your hair, you need to understand the concept of ionic bonding.

Substances that have a negative charge are called anionic. Substances that have a zero charge are called non-ionic. Substances that have a positive charge are called cationic. Substances that have both positive and negative charges are called zwitterionic.

The ingredients in shampoos and conditioners are formulated with different charges to help them interact and bind with the proteins on the hair fiber—specifically, on the cuticle. The interaction of the charges of the ingredients in shampoo and conditioner with the charge of the hair is referred to as ionic interaction. Shampoos are formulated so that they can be rinsed off the hair, and conditioners are formulated so that they stay on the hair.

Most of the time, hair is anionic, which means that it has a negative charge. Sometimes, however, hair can be non-ionic, which means that it has a zero charge. In layman's terms, damaged hair has a more negative charge than healthy hair. It's thirsty and it loves water. A material or surface that loves water is called hydrophilic.

Hair care products, especially conditioners, are formulated to address the needs of damaged hair. This may seem like a contradiction, because many of us have healthy hair and just use shampoos and conditioners to maintain it. That is true, but as long as your hair is on your head, it is always moving toward a damaged state. Everything you do to your hair, including keeping it immobilized, washing it or even touching it, can potentially damage your hair. Thus, hair care products are made for hair that is assumed to be already damaged or moving toward being damaged.

Some conditioning products are formulated to spread well and deposit uniformly on the more damaged hair. These products will usually contain positively charged, or cationic, ingredients. Positive is attracted to negative: the positively charged ingredients in a hair conditioner are attracted to the most negatively charged areas on the surface of the hair.

Shampoos and Conditioners: General Characteristics

Shampoos

Shampoos are made to remove dirt, particles and grease from the hair. In general, they are formulated to have a negative charge. In other words, shampoos tend to be anionic. The surfactant molecules that make up shampoos have a head that is attracted to water and a tail that is attracted to dirt. Shampoos contain ingredients that are attracted to water, so that when the hair is rinsed, the shampoo leaves the hair. When the shampoo is rinsed away, the ingredients in the shampoo pull dirt and oil away from the hair strands and scalp.

It is not the foaming ingredient in the shampoo that strips the dirt and oil. The ingredient that strips the dirt is called a surfactant. Foam is placed in the shampoo because the average consumer believes that shampoo must foam in order to function properly. This is part of the marketing aspect of hair care products. Foaming ingredients are added to create foam, not to clean.

Conditioners

In general, conditioners are formulated with positive charges. In other words, they tend to be cationic. This means that they are formulated to be attracted to the hair and coat hair that is damaged. The positively charged conditioners are attracted to the most negatively charged part of the hair strand, which is the most damaged part, and they will coat and bind to it.

Whether a store-bought hair care product is a shampoo or a conditioner, it will contain only three main types of components or ingredients:

1. Solvent (usually water)
2. Surfactant, or a system of surfactants
3. Additives

Surfactant stands for "surface active agent." Surfactants are the workhorses in shampoos and conditioners. Most commercial shampoos, conditioners and other hair care products are made primarily of surfactants. Surfactants perform four functions: cleansing, foaming, wetting and emulsifying. Later, we will look at each function separately.

What Shampoo Does to Your Hair

The surfactant in the shampoo interacts with the protein of the cuticle. A common surfactant in shampoos is sodium laureth sulfate, or SLS. This surfactant binds with the proteins in the endocuticle. The endocuticle is a sheet-like subcomponent of the cuticle. The proteins in the endocuticle do not have any chemical disulfide bonds. They are held together instead by ionic links with an overall negative charge.

SLS is negatively charged, or anionic. Since similar charges repel each other, when the SLS binds to the hair, the endocuticle, which is also negatively charged, swells to repel the SLS. This is one reason why the SLS doesn't stay bound to the hair; it washes out once water is applied.

Thus the SLS causes a reaction in the endocuticle that makes the cuticle lift or swell. When you have shampooed your hair and you stop to feel it before you condition it, the hair surface feels rougher than it did before you washed it. What you are feeling is the result of the charge repulsion on the hair because of the surfactant. All the negative charges are trying to get away from the other negative charges, or pulling away from one another. The result is the lifted cuticle. In addition to lifting or roughening the cuticle in this way, SLS also degrades or removes protein from the hair. For these reasons, many people prefer to not use products which contain sulfates (sulphates), or SLS.

What Conditioner Does to Your Hair

The surfactant in the conditioner also binds to the endocuticle. A common ingredient in conditioners is quaternary ammonium salts. They are cationic, or positively charged. They also contain certain components that are hydrophobic, which means they are afraid of or dislike water.

When these surfactants get on the hair, their positive charge is attracted to the negative charge of the hair. Because of this ionic bonding, one part of these surfactants stays on the hair even after the hair has been rinsed. Because of their hydrophobic components, however, another part of the surfactant tries to get away from the water used to rinse the hair. So the molecules of the surfactant have one end that is attached to the hair and another end that hangs from the hair, unattached. The unbound, hanging ends of the surfactant combine with the unbound, hanging ends of other surfactants from the same solution. As the surfactants combine with each other and get away from the water, they contract. This causes the cuticle to de-swell and lie down flatter along the hair strand, creating a smooth surface on the hair. In reality, the hair surface has not changed, but the way it feels has changed. These surfactants function like a new, smooth surface on the hair. This smooth surface is temporary. It lasts only until the surfactant is removed.

How to Use Conditioners Effectively

Conditioners are formulated to have maximum effectiveness after approximately three cycles. This means that before you judge whether a conditioning product works for you, use it about once a week for at least three weeks. By the third or fourth week, you should know whether the product is working for you. You cannot apply a conditioner only one time and expect it to continue to work forever after that one application. Whenever you try a new conditioner, try to use it for about three cycles, or about three weeks, to know if it is working for you. This is a general rule.

Important Points to Know about Conditioners

Conditioners work on the surface of the hair.

You, the consumer, are paying attention to the surface of your hair. Therefore, most hair care products are designed to work on the surface of the hair. Thus, the purpose of a conditioner is to improve the surface of the hair.

The effects of conditioners are temporary.

This means that they must be applied over and over to continue to affect the surface of the hair.

Product build-up should be removed periodically.

This is because you want the product to work directly with the hair strand. You don't want the product to be blocked by or to bind with old product that has been left on the hair.

Conditioners can't repair hair.

Even if a conditioner is marketed with claims that it can repair hair damage, the reality is that they cannot repair damage permanently. What conditioners can do is make your hair feel as if it has been repaired. This is because conditioners act upon the surface of the hair. They make the hair look and feel different from the way it did before you used them. Cosmetic companies can say that their conditioning products repair hair because these products simulate the look and feel of hair that has been repaired, but the effect is temporary.

Conditioners make hair easier to comb.

Conditioners are formulated to make hair easier to comb. They provide lubrication to both wet and dry hair.

Conditioners reduce the charges from the two types of electricity on the hair.

As mentioned, there are two types of electric conductivity on the hair: triboelectricity, which comes from rubbing one hair against another, and piezoelectricity, which comes from pressure, as when you press down on your hair with a comb or brush.

Flyaway hair is a result of triboelectricity. Damaged hair tends to be more negatively charged than healthy hair. When two negatively charged hairs meet, they repel each other. This makes them stand away from each other. When the individual strands of hair are standing away from each other, this creates what is called flyaway hair.

When you place conditioner, which contains positively charged ingredients, on the negatively charged hair, the conditioner bonds with the hair. This temporarily reduces the hair's negative charge. The result is that the hairs are not pushing away from one another, and flyaway hairs are reduced. And when you place conditioner on the hair and then comb or brush it, the pull or pressure from the styling implement is lessened by the presence of the conditioner. There is less friction, and the comb or brush can slide through the hair more easily, with less pressure.

Product ingredients are constantly increasing and changing. New chemicals are synthesized every day. There is no way I can create an exhaustive, up-to-date list. My purpose is to give you a general idea, so that you know what to look for and how to categorize an ingredient in a hair product.

I mentioned earlier that most shampoos and conditioners contain three kinds of ingredients. These are solvents; surfactants, or a system of surfactants; and additives. Let's talk about these in detail. I think you are ready now!

Solvents

Solvents are liquids that serve as carriers for other ingredients. They evaporate after the product has been applied to the hair. Solvents are usually water-based. Solvents are also referred to as plasticizing agents. These are ingredients that coat a surface and make it smooth. Some other ingredients, such as panthenol, aloe vera and silicone, also work as plasticizers but are not considered solvents. You are not trying to become a cosmetic chemist, so you don't have to get stuck in these details.

I like to divide the solvents into four main groups: water, alcohol, glycol, and miscellaneous.

Water

Water is considered a universal solvent. It is used to dissolve many things. Usually, water is the first ingredient listed on a shampoo or conditioner bottle. You may see different types of water specified.

- Distilled–distilled water has been heat-treated to remove impurities. It is sometimes called dead water because the positively and negatively charged components within the water have been removed.
- De-ionized–de-ionized water is similar to distilled water.
- Spring water–spring water is supposed to be water that comes from a spring. We can assume, though, that it has come out of a tap or faucet and not from a mountaintop somewhere.
- Sea water–sea water may have come from the sea, or it may simulate sea water by containing salt, seaweed or other marine components.

Don't let these names dazzle or confuse you. Just know that the first ingredient in your shampoo or conditioner is probably some form of water.

Alcohol

There are four types of alcohol that you are likely to find used as solvents: SD alcohol, isopropyl alcohol, benzyl alcohol, and lauryl alcohol. We don't need to define these. Just be able to recognize them on the label of your products.

SD stands for "specially denatured," which is alcohol that is not intended for human consumption. This means that you should not drink it. It is not likely that you will see isopropyl alcohol in many of your hair products. You never know, though. Technically, lauryl alcohol is not a solvent but a controller of viscosity, or thickness.

Glycol

Another type of solvent is glycol-based. You recognize these by the end of the name. All glycol-based solvent names end in "lene +glycol." Here are some examples of glycol solvents: propylene glycol, hexylene glycol, butylene glycol, dipropylene glycol, and octylene glycol. You can look them up at your leisure, if you like. The purpose here is just to be able to recognize and categorize these ingredients, so you know what you are using on your hair.

Miscellaneous

Some other types of solvents you may find in your hair products are acetamide MEA, glycerine, tallow poly amine (PEG-#), methylene chloride, phenoxyethanol, sulfated castor oil, mineral oil, and polysorbate.

Surfactants

Surfactants in General

Surfactant stands for "surface active agent." Surfactants are the workhorses in shampoos and conditioners. Most commercial shampoos and conditioners are made up of 70%-90% surfactants. They contain not just one surfactant but a system of surfactants.

Surfactants can perform four different functions: cleansing, foaming, wetting or emulsifying. We will look at each function separately.

Cleansing

The average shampoo contains at least one anionic, or negatively charged, surfactant. Cationic, or positively charged, surfactants are also used in shampoos, but they are more luxurious and more expensive. Cationic surfactants are usually used in shampoos for their antimicrobial properties.

Because cationic or positively charged surfactants bind to the hair, they are used in conditioners. They are not in there for cleansing and foaming because they cost too much; something cheaper can be used for these two functions. Cationic or positively charged surfactants are modified chemically so that they do not combine with anionic surfactants to form a substance that is solid. Two surfactants combined unintentionally with one another can't help your hair. That's because they bind with one another and not your hair. Once they bind with one another, this renders them ineffective.

Foaming

Foam in shampoos is generated by excess surfactant. Foam does not cleanse the hair. Consumers believe that the more something foams, the better it's working, so cosmetics companies accommodate you and make their shampoos foam. Surfactants that foam tend to be anionic, or negatively charged.

Wetting

Some surfactants are used to make a product wetter. These types of surfactants are mostly found in conditioners. They are usually water soluble, which means that they dissolve in water. They are used to dissolve a powder that might not dissolve if it was placed directly in water.

Emulsifying/Dispersing

These types of surfactants are used to bind ingredients, such as oil and water, in a product. Surfactants used for emulsifying are usually nonionic. They have no charge, so they are compatible with both positively charged and negatively charged ingredients.

Surfactants can be ranked in order of harshness. Surfactants with a zero charge, or non-ionics, tend to be mildest. Surfactants with a negative (-) charge are mild, and surfactants with a positive (+) charge tend to be the harshest. Cationic, or positively charged, surfactants are usually used in a product to condition the hair.

Surfactants in Detail

Surfactants are like bulldogs. They go after any and all grime, dirt and oil on a surface. Surfactants can't distinguish between oil that is dirt and oil that is essential for the lubrication and proper care of the hair. Thus, when using a shampoo that contains surfactants, you may have to return oil to the hair by adding oil or some fatty material to your hair.

Soap is a surfactant. Regular soap can ruin the hair. Soap makes the proteins in the hair swell, and then leaches or pulls them from the hair. This can cause the hair to deteriorate very quickly if the soap is not thoroughly rinsed away. Hair feels rougher after you have used soap on it.

Breaking Down Surfactants by Charge and Type

Technically, there are four types of surfactants: anionic, nonionic, cationic and amphoteric. Let's look at each in more detail. These are types of substances. As a point of clarification and as a reminder, there are four types of charges: anionic, nonionic, cationic and zwitterionic. Zwitterionic refers to substances with both a negative and positive charge. Amphoteric refers to a substance or compound that can act either as an acid or a base.

Anionic (Foaming and cleansing type)

Most anionic, or negatively charged, substances are used for foaming and cleansing. An anionic surfactant is usually the primary type of surfactant found in shampoos. Anionic surfactants are found in other hair care products as well, including conditioners and protein treatment products.

Look at the list below. You want to be able to recognize these ingredients on the back of the bottle and know what category they fall into.

- sulfates
- sulfonates
- carboxylates (soap falls into this category)
- phosphates and amides

These are four common types of anionic surfactants that can be found in shampoos and conditioners. Most people are familiar with sulfates; some try to avoid them. Sulfate-free shampoos are becoming more popular and easy to find.

Non-Ionic (primary support type)

Non-ionic surfactants are those that have no charge. Many non-ionic surfactants are found in shampoos. They are not the main cleaning ingredient in a shampoo, but are used to support the primary surfactant. Some of their name endings are "oxide," "ester," and "xylate." Look for:

- alkanolamides (may end in "oxide")
- esters
- ethyloxylates
- propoxylates

Cationic (conditioning and cleansing type)

Cationic surfactants have a positive charge. Cationic surfactants are what do the work in hair products. Again, you want to familiarize yourself with these to be able to quickly identify them and categorize them when you see them listed among product ingredients.

- quaternary ammonium compounds
- amines

Amphoteric (detoxifying or irritation-minimizing type)

Amphoteric surfactants may go from a positive to a negative charge when there is a change in the pH. A more acidic or more basic ingredient added to the formulation could cause a change in the pH. If the environment or solution around an amphoteric substance is more acidic, the amphoteric substance will become more acidic. If the environment or solution around the amphoteric substance is basic, the amphoteric substance will become basic. Thus, amphoterics are not usually used, and it is not likely that you will see an amphoteric listed on your bottle. You never know, though! Four examples of these types of surfactants are:

- imidazolene
- betaines
- sultaines

Additives

Shampoos and conditioner contain many types of additives. Let's discuss some of the ones you might see most frequently.

Conditioning Agents

Conditioning agents fall into three categories: surfactants, proteins, and fatty or oily materials. We have already discussed surfactants, and we will come to fatty materials in the section on lubrication. Let's look at proteins as conditioning agents.

Protein hydrolysates (also called polypeptides)

Proteins are conditioning agents. Protein is very important for Afro-textured hair because it helps to fortify or strengthen a damaged or weakened hair strand. Proteins also can re-texturize the surface of your hair strand and make it feel smoother in the sense that it fills in cracks and missing cuticle layers. Proteins are more useful in conditioners than in shampoos. They impart manageability to the hair. They add shine and gloss because they smooth the surface which makes the hair strand better able to capture and reflect light. Proteins are more effective if left on the hair for a while longer than if they are rinsed off immediately.

A hydrolysate is simply a substance that has been broken down into a size smaller than its original size. Conversely, a condensate is a molecule that has been built up. Condensates are usually found in shampoos, and hydrolysates are found in conditioners. Here are some characteristics of hydrolysates:

- They form a film on a surface, such as your hair, without smothering it;
- They bind to water to help a surface, such as the hair, enhance its ability to absorb and maintain water;
- They break down in water.
- They are especially effective on bleached or damaged hair.

Types of Protein Hydrolysates

There are three kinds of protein hydrolysates: marine, animal and plant. This is just a fancy way to say that there are three categories of proteins for your hair. All proteins are made up of amino acids. It is the sequence or order of the amino acids within the protein that determines the type of protein. Protein hydrolysates can penetrate the hair strand and deposit in the cortex.

Marine

Marine protein hydrolysates are derived from the sea. They can come from red, green or blue algae and kelp, or they can be derived from careegan, which is also known as Irish moss. Other kinds of marine protein are seaweed, chlorella and spirullina.

Animal

Animal protein hydrolysates are derived from animals. These sources tend to be the least expensive and most commonly used. Some ways you may see these listed on your labels are as animal protein, silk from worms, cholesterol, keratin amino acids, elastin, yeast and casein from cow's milk. Collagen is an animal protein, but it is not a protein hydrolysate; it is a complete protein.

Plant

Plant hydrolysates are derived from plants. Although seaweed and algae are plants, they fit into the Marine category and not this one. Some examples of plant protein hydrolysates that you may see in a list of ingredients are soy, wheat, vegetable, pea and corn.

Amino Acids

Amino acids are constituents of protein. Amino acids such as cysteine, cystine and tryptophan are very water soluble and can sometimes be considered hygroscopic, which means that they attract water. They can penetrate the hair shaft and help the hair to maintain a good moisture balance. Amino acids are related to protein hydrolysates because all proteins are made up of amino acids

Humectants, or Hygroscopic Conditioning Agents

Another category of conditioning agents is humectants. Humectants are used to attract water to a surface or substance. A fancy word for something that attracts water is hygroscopic. Humectants place a film on the hair that is occlusive, or somewhat smothering. This film lubricates the hair and stops it from losing moisture. There are about three common categories of humectants: amino acids, sugars (also called saccharides), and protein hydrosylates. Glycerin is also a humectant. Here is a list of some humectants:

- amino acids
  - taurine
  - cysteine
  - cysteine
  - methionine

- sugars (saccharides)
  - muccopolysaccharides
  - honey
  - guar gum

- protein hydrolysates
- glycerin
- allaintoin

Lubricating Substances

Lubricants coat the hair and can form a film on the hair. Listed below are some categories of lubricating substances. They differ from humectants in that they help the hairs to move smoothly across one another by reducing friction on the hair.

- fatty material
- fatty alcohols
- silicones
- water
- panthenol
- aloe vera

Fatty Material as Lubricants

There are two categories of fatty material. One category is natural oil. This includes but is not limited to olive oil, coconut oil, sesame oil and jojoba oil. Technically, jojoba is a wax, but it still provides lubrication. A second category of fatty material is hydrocarbons. Hydrocarbons are synthesized from petroleum oil. Two common hydrocarbons that are used as lubricants are mineral oil and petrolatum. Here are some names of fatty material to look for:

⊘ natural oils
⊘ hydrocarbons
  ○ mineral oil
  ○ petrolatum
  ○ paraffin
  ○ squalane

Fatty Alcohols as Lubricants

Fatty alcohols are also used as lubricants in hair products. Fatty alcohols are derived from plant and animal oils and fats. Look for the ingredients on this list and be able to identify them.

⊘ cetearyl alcohol
⊘ cetyl alcohol
⊘ stearyl alcohol
⊘ lauryl alcohol

Silicones as Lubricants

Silicone does not prevent moisture from leaving or entering the hair strand. Although silicones are not occlusive, meaning they do not smoother the hair strand, they can be difficult to remove, even with clarifying shampoos.

There are two kinds of silicones: volatile and substantive. Volatile silicones are formulated for the benefit of wet hair. They help wet hair to feel smooth. They are designed to provide lubrication as a middle, or temporary, stage in the washing and conditioning process. Once the hair dries, these types of silicones have performed their job. Substantive silicones are formulated to provide slip and lubrication for dry hair. Unlike the volatile silicones, they do not evaporate or disappear. The volatile silicones are transitory or temporary, while the substantive silicones stick around—literally.

If your product directions suggest that you use the product on wet hair and you see silicones in the list of ingredients, you can assume that the product contains volatile silicones. If the directions suggest that you use the product on dry hair and you see silicones in the list, you can assume that the product contains substantive silicones.

You can recognize silicone in two ways. The easiest way is that the name will end in "cone." You may also see silicones that end in "oxane." Here are some examples of silicones that you may see on product labels:

- cyclopentasiloxane
- amodimethicone
- cyclomethicone
- dimethicone
- dimethicone copolyol
- simethicone
- stearoxydimethicone

Cyclopentasiloxane is often found in skin care products and make-up. It is also found in some hair care products. Dimethicone is one of the most commonly used silicone products in the personal care industry. Simethicone is used as an anti-foaming agent.

Color

Color is another additive in hair care products. Colors can be natural or synthetic. Some examples are listed below.

Natural Colors

- henna, henna extract
- carotene
- titanium dioxide
- zinc oxide
- mica
- betonite

Synthetic Colors

- FD & C
- D & C

⌣ caramel
⌣ disodium EDTA copper

Fragrance

Fragrance is one of the easiest additives to identify. Usually, the ingredient list will have the word "fragrance." Extracts, oils and synthetic perfumes are just a few of the many substances that can be used to scent a product.

If a product is sold in Europe it must comply with the European Union Cosmetic Directive. This mandate requires that all hair products in Europe list the components of their fragrance, from a total of 27 specified in the mandate. I have listed the most commonly used. By the way, these ingredients can also be found in perfumes and toilet water.

⌣ benzyl salicytate (fragrance stabilizer)
⌣ limonene
⌣ citral
⌣ citronellol
⌣ coumarine
⌣ eugenol
⌣ geraniol
⌣ linalool
⌣ A isomethyl ionone
⌣ amyl cinnamal
⌣ benzyl alcohol
⌣ benzyl benzoate
⌣ farmesol
⌣ hexylcinnamal
⌣ hydroxy cintronellal
⌣ lyral

Preservatives and Anti-Microbials

Preservatives, which are usually water based, are placed in a product to stop the growth of bacteria or fungi. Preservatives are used in hair conditioners that have a comparatively large number of additives.

The main purpose of the preservatives is to protect the product, not your hair. They are used to preserve the shelf life of a product.

Preservatives

Preservatives are divided into two groups: bactericides and fungicides. Bactericides are active against bacteria, and fungicides are active against fungi, yeast and molds.

- ◯ bactericide
    - ○ myrstalkonium chloride
- ◯ fungicides
    - ○ DMDM hydantoin
    - ○ disodium EDTA
    - ○ terasodium EDTA
    - ○ dimethyl ether
    - ○ benzophenone-N
    - ○ sodium sulfite
    - ○ sulfur
    - ○ methylisothiazolinone
    - ○ methylchloroisthiazolinone

Anti-Microbials

Anti-microbial ingredients are used in hair conditioners. Their job is to inhibit the growth of micro-organisms or destroy them. The categories of anti-microbial components to look for are formaldehyde, phenolics or parabens, alcohols, acids, chlorine compounds, quaternary ammonium compounds and fatty acids.

- ◯ formadelhyde
    - ○ hydontoin
    - ○ urea
- ◯ phenolics/ parabens
    - ○ methyl paraben
    - ○ propyl paraben
    - ○ butyl paraben

- alcohols
- acids
    - benzoic acid
    - sorbic acid
    - salicyc acid

- chlorine compounds
- quaternary ammonium compounds

    - quartenium 14
    - quartenium 15

- fatty acids (end in "mide")
    - acetamide MEA
    - lauramide MIPA
    - oleamide MIPA

pH Adjusters and pH Controllers

Other additives in hair care products are pH adjusters and pH controllers. Some ingredients have both a positive and a negative charge. Depending on the pH, the substance may change to a positively charged or a negatively charged substance.

Also, product formulators want to ensure that the products do not irritate the body tissues of the consumer. Thus, it is important that all products be placed in a safe pH range. The pH adjusters and controllers ensure that solutions are not too alkaline or too acidic.

- apple cider vinegar
- disodium phosphate
- EDTA
- acids
    - boric acid
    - adipic acid
    - citric acid
    - formic acid
    - glycolic acid
    - lactic acid

o   hydrochloric acid

o   phosphoric acid

◎ sodium hydroxide

I have seen sodium hydroxide listed as an ingredient in deep conditioners for frizzy or curly hair. If you have natural hair that you want to keep in a natural state, you may want to remain vigilant regarding this ingredient. If it is listed on the label, that means it comprises at least 1% of the product. Some people believe this concentration is so small that it is not significant, but a product can be considered a relaxer if it has 1% sodium hydroxide. If this ingredient appears on the list, the possibility exists that it may be present in sufficient quantity to chemically alter and straighten your natural hair. You need to make your own decision. If you don't have the information, the decision is made for you.

Thickeners and Viscosity Adjusters

Thickeners and viscosity adjusters are used to make a hair care product creamier and less runny. Viscosity relates to the flow of a fluid. The faster the fluid flows, the lower the viscosity. The higher the viscosity, the slower the fluid flows. Thickeners are also defined as thickening agents, emulsifying agents and stabilizers. Some of the common categories of thickeners are polysaccharides, gums and resins.

Polysaccharides

Polysaccharides dissolve in water. Corn starch, pectin and cellulose are thickeners that fall into the polysaccharide category. Aloe vera has a component that makes it a polysaccharide. Remember, many ingredients can fall into one or more categories.

Gums

Technically, gums are polysaccharides but we will place them in their own category. There are two major kinds of gums: marine and non-marine. Algin and carrageenan (Irish moss) are marine gums.

Gum Arabic, guar gum and gum tracanath come from trees and plants. Xanthum gum is synthesized from fermented sugar.

Resins

Resins come from plants. Resins do not dissolve in water. They do dissolve in oil, though. Sandalwood oil and balsam are examples of resins. Resins have strong scents and can be used for scenting and thickening a product.

Other Thickeners

Other types of thickeners are clays, psyllium husks and hyaluronic acid. Carbomers are synthetic thickeners. Carbomers are often found in gels.

- Polysaccharides
    - corn starch
    - pectin
    - cellulose
    - aloe vera

- Gums
    - marine gums
        - algin
        - carrageenan
    - plant or tree gums
        - gum arabic
        - gum traganath
        - guar gum
    - xanthum gum

- Resins
    - balsam
    - benzoin gum
    - sandalwood oil

⟲ Other
- o natural clays (betonite)
- o psyllium husk
- o hyaluronic acid (hydrolyzed mucopolysaccharide)
- o carbomer (acrylic acid)

Viscosity Adjusters

There are many kinds of viscosity adjusters and controllers. Silica, sodium chloride, ammonium chloride, SD alcohol (ethyl alcohol) and lecithin are considered viscosity adjusters.

Some surfactants are used as viscosity adjusters. There are so many of them that it is just easier to stick surfactants in the surfactant category. Most of the time, I don't recognize surfactants by sight. Usually, I identify what might be a surfactant by elimination. I will be able to identify many of the other components first. Usually, whatever component is left over falls into the surfactant category. Surfactants are hard enough to try to identify. Don't worry about surfactants being used as a viscosity controller or adjuster.

Herbs and Vitamins

Herbs and vitamins can also be listed as additives in a hair care product. I am not going to list them here, as the list would be endless. Also, many of you are familiar with your favorite herbs and vitamins.

The amount of herbs and vitamins in the average product is minimal. I have read that herbs and vitamins don't make a difference for your hair. I don't agree with this. I do believe that the amount of herbs and vitamins present in most commercially made, store-bought products don't make a difference for your hair. This is not because the herbs and vitamins don't provide benefits, it's because there is not enough of them in the average product to impart those benefits.

If you are making your own products, you control the amount of herbs and vitamins that go into the product. I believe that herbs and vitamins can penetrate the hair and scalp and do good things for your hair. The key is in their quantity and formulation. I will discuss vitamins and herbs for your hair, as well as other ideas, in my next hair book. There's just not enough space and time in the present book.

Protein Treatments and Reconstruction Treatments

Two more product types are important for you to understand: protein treatments and reconstructors. Many products available today use these two words interchangeably for the same types of products. I like to make a distinction between the two products. My distinction is not necessarily scientific. It has to do with the way these products are marketed.

For a product to be considered a protein treatment, the purpose of the product should be to improve the look and feel of the hair, or to make the surface of the hair strand smoother. The result from the use of the protein treatment should be smoother, shinier, glossier hair.

For a product to be considered a reconstructor, the purpose of the product should be to repair split ends. This product focuses on the tip of the hair strand. After you use a reconstructor, it is the ends of your hair that should be smoother, less frizzy, silkier, healthier. You should not see split ends.

Both types of products give the appearance that the hair has been repaired, but neither one actually repairs hair permanently. The action of both products is purely temporary. As you know, the reality is that once the hair structure has been damaged, no product can repair it.

How to Get the Most from Treatments and Products

Before moving to the treatments, two important concepts must be clear in your mind so that you can understand the difference between protein treatments and reconstructors. The two concepts are adsorption and absorption, and the best types of heat to use for each.

Adsorption and Absorption

Adsorption is when a product binds to the surface of a substance. Adsorption occurs on the outside of the hair strand, on the cuticle of the hair, when you use conditioners. Conditioning rinses are formulated to bind to the very top or the surface of the hair. Most inexpensive conditioning rinses are not intended to penetrate into the hair. Components in the conditioner are positively charged and bind with the negatively charged surface of the hair.

Absorption occurs when a product penetrates the surface of a substance. Water can be absorbed into hair: it penetrates the hair strand and reaches the cortex of the hair.

Dry Heat and Wet Heat

Dry heat occurs in the traditional use of a hot air dryer. Dry heat is air that has been warmed and then blown on the hair. This type of heat comes from the standard blow dryer and from the hooded dryers that are often seen in beauty salons. Generally, this type of heat contains no moisture or water.

Wet heat is moist, hot air or steam. Steam heat is created when water is warmed to the point of vaporization and is then blown onto the hair. You can get this type of heat by wetting your hair and placing a hot, wet towel over it. You can also experience this type of heat by using an apparatus such as a hair steamer.

Adsorption and Dry Heat

As already stated, adsorption occurs when a product or ingredient binds or sticks to the surface of another substance. If you are using a product that is meant to address the surface of your hair, such as protein or rinse-off conditioner, my suggestion would be to use dry, hot air for best results. Why? If you use hot air or dry heat, the water in the product evaporates, leaving the active components to bind to the hair.

Absorption and Wet Heat

Absorption occurs when a product or ingredient penetrates the surface of a substance and enters the interior of that substance. If you are using a product that is meant to impact the inner component of your hair, my suggestion would be to use wet air for best results. Why? If you use wet heat, the hair strand swells and the cuticle is raised. This allows the water in the product to penetrate the hair with ease and carry the active ingredients of the product to the inside of the strand.

Protein Treatments and Reconstructors in Detail

Protein Treatments

In general, protein treatments contain larger, positively charged or cationic components or molecules. They are often broken down or hydrolyzed to be made smaller than their original natural size in order to better attach to the hair. These positively charged components bind to the negatively charged surface of the hair. Remember, damaged hair is more negatively charged than healthier hair. Therefore, the components of the treatment will gravitate to the more damaged parts of the hair.

Protein treatments are formulated to adsorb, or bind to the surface of the hair. Therefore, if you want to obtain the maximum benefits of these products, you may want to use them with hot air or dry heat.

Reconstructor Treatments

In general, reconstructor treatments contain components or molecules that are smaller in size, that are both positively and negatively charged. These charged components penetrate the hair strand. They are meant to concentrate in the inner components of the hair strand, such as the cortex.

In the case of a damaged cuticle, the hair surface may be chipped, the cuticle may be missing completely, or there may be microscopic breaks or fissures on the strand. In the case of a split hair, the cortex has been damaged. The result is that the inner part of the hair has been split into two sections. This type of break is what is called a split end. The needs of split ends, which indicate a splitting of the cortex, are different from the needs of the hair cuticle that has cracks on the surface. A split hair has been damaged at its core. It will not respond to being coated by a product. A cracked hair, or a hair with a missing cuticle or a roughened, dull surface, will have a better appearance after being coated by a product.

Reconstructors, or split end repair treatments, contain extra-small and extra-large proteins to fill in cracks and ruptured areas on and inside the hair shaft. They may also contain components to bind the split pieces of the cortex together. These products are formulated to be absorbed into the hair.

Inside the wet hair strand, the particles of the product components break down. Some of the particles are positively charged, and some are negatively charged. The particles distribute themselves on both sides of the split cortex, with both positively and negatively charged particles on each side. The positively charged components on each side of the cortex become attracted to the negatively charged components on the other side. The opposite charges "reach out" to each other across the split. This makes the charged particles form a bridge across the split hair, which pulls the split hairs back into place. The result is the appearance of repaired split ends. The hair no longer appears to be split. In reality, it is still split. The split will become apparent when the product wears off of or is washed from the hair.

In addition to this bridging action, another component, such as an acrylic or vinyl type ingredient, is placed in the product that binds and holds the hair together once the product dries. This will help to keep the split hairs bound together, temporarily until the hair is washed again.

If you want to obtain the maximum benefit of this type of recontstructor treatment, you may want to use it with wet or steamed heat. This will allow for maximum penetration of the product into the hair strand or cortex. In addition to applying the product with wet heat, you may want to follow up with dry heat. The dry heat will facilitate the evaporation of the water from the product, leaving behind the components that are intended to bind to the hair. This will help the protein to deposit or stay on the hair strand. It will also help the two pieces of the split hair to stay stuck together.

Dry heat	Wet heat
Best for protein treatments.	Best for reconstructor treatments.
Sit under a dryer with protein treatments until hair has become less damp.	Cover wet head with a cap, and use with or without external heat. Or sit under a hair steamer.
Uses adsorbtion, which pertains to binding or sticking to a surface, which is the cuticle.	Uses absorption, which pertains to penetrating or going inside a substance's surface, to the cortex.
Protein treatments deposit on the outside hair.	Reconstructor treatments deposit inside the hair.
Protein treatments work to coat the hair and provide shine and gloss. They help with making the hair easier to comb.	Reconstructor treatments work to strengthen the inner part or cortex of the hair.
Protein affects the feel and the texture of the surface of the cuticle of the hair.	Bind split hairs together on a strand by strand basis.
Use drying agents and ionic bonding to attach to the surface of the hair.	Use resins and acrylics to stick the hairs together. Use ionic bonding, or bridging to re-join split hairs.

Product Type	Shampoo	Conditioner
Solvent	Water-based, alcohol-based	Water based, alcohol- based
Surfactants	Surfactant for cleansing and for foaming. Usually negatively charged.	Surfactant for coating and lubricating the hair. Usually positively charged.
Additives	Conditioning agents	Conditioning agents
	Active ingredients (as in dandruff shampoos)	Bridging agents to help the conditioner ingredients to hind stronger to the hair
	Opacifiers or opaque, shiny looking ingredients	Oily or waxy substances to lubricate the hair strand
	color	color
	fragrance	fragrance
	preservatives	preservatives
	pH adjusters	pH adjusters
	Thickeners, also called viscosity builders	Thickeners, also called viscosity builders

In Closing

You will never know every single component in a store-bought cosmetic. Any ingredient that comprises less than 1% of the product doesn't have to be listed, and listed ingredients that comprise only a small percentage can be named in any order.

In addition, new chemicals are synthesized every day. There is no way that you can keep up with all the names and product types. You don't really need to know them, though. All you need is a basic idea of the common components and ingredients in hair care products. Your purpose is not to recreate the product, but to ensure that you are getting the best product for your hair. You want to be able to select your products based upon knowledge, not just marketing. This will empower you.

With the knowledge you have gained from this book, you can focus on products that will help you, rather than on products that seem magical. When you look for magic, you can become disillusioned and disappointed. You can't afford this any more than you can afford to waste your money. You have more important things to feel, and more important things to spend your money on. Whatever you do and whatever you buy, spend your life energy and your money wisely.

CHAPTER 8

Step 4: Putting It All Together

Cheat Sheets

Do you like cheat sheets? They are tools to help support a process. I suggest that you copy this chart, stick it in your purse or bag and take it with you. That way, when you run across a product, you can whip out the chart and do some quick, high-level analysis on the product before you buy it.

As I said at the beginning, I am not telling you which products or ingredients are good for you and which are bad for you. That's your job. I have given you a process and the tools to help you identify, recognize and categorize the ingredients. This will help you determine whether a product might be right for you. Then you can use the product and determine which ingredients in it may be working as you hoped they would and which may not.

You have to continue to get familiar with this information and practice using it. If you are taught by a person who understands her subject and knows how to teach it, you can understand anything, including rocket science.

Category 1: Solvents Cheat Sheet

Group Name	Pattern/How to Identify It	Examples of It	Usual/ Common Location on Label	Notes
Water	Ends in "water"	Water, distilled, de-ionized, agua, aqua, eau, sea water, marine water, spring water, purified water	Near top of ingredient list	
Alcohol	Ends in "alcohol"	SD alcohol, iso-propyl alcohol, benzyl alcohol, lauryl alcohol	Near top or middle of ingredient list	SD stands for "specifically de-natured alcohol." Alcohol for consumption is usually ethanol. SD alcohol can sometimes be followed by a number (SD al-cohol 40)
Glycol	Ends in "lene + glycol"	Propylene glycol, hexylene glycol, butylene glycol, glyceryl	Near top or middle of ingre-dient list	
Miscella-neous	No pattern	Acetamide MEA, Glycerine, PEG-#, Methy-lene chloride, phenoxyethanol, sulfated castor oil, polysorbate		The PEG ingredient can be followed by various numbers.

Category 2: Surfactants Cheat Sheet

Group Name	Pattern/How to Identify It	Examples of It	Ususal/Common Location on Label	Notes
Anionic	Ending in: Sulfate Sulfonate Phosphate		Top	Found in shampoos. Tend to be used for **cleansing**. Tend to be used for **foaming** as in to make foam.
Non-Ionic (Supports the primary surfactant in the formula)	Fatty alcohols Ending In: "glucoside" "yl + alcohol" "Ceteareth + #" "Steareth + #" Glyceryl stearate Look for words with glycol in the middle	Cocoglucaside, capryl gluco-side, Cetyl alcohol, stearyl alcohol, ceteostearyl alcohol, oleyl alcohol, Ceteareth -20 Cocomide DEA, Cocomide MEA	Top to middle	Found in conditioners. Tend to be used for **emulsifying** or dispersing Tend to be used for **wetting**. Fatty alcohols are non-ionic surfactants but I have them listed in the additive section, under alcohols.
Cationic (Conditioning)	Quaternary Ammonium compounds ending in "ium + chloride" "ium + bromide" "amine"		Top to middle	Found in conditioners. Tend to be used to **condition** or improve the surface feel of the hair.
Zwitter-ionic/Am-photeric	Look for words that end in: "Amino acids" "Betaine" "Sultaine" Lecithin Imidazoline derivatives		Middle	In general, found in shampoos. Amino acids are often found in conditioners, though. Tend to be used to **detoxify**, meaning to minimize the irritation of other ingredients.

Category 3: Additives Cheat Sheet				
Group Name	Pattern/How to Identify It	Examples of It	Usual/Common Location on Label	Notes
Protein Hydroly-sates: Animal		Keratin amino acids, silk, elastin, yeast, casein, gelatin, protein	Depends on product	Collagen is a complete protein, not a protein hy-droslysate. They are also referred to as polypep-tides.
Protein Hydro-lysates: Plant	Proteins from plants and veg-etables that are land based	Soy, wheat, veg-etable, pea, corn	Depends on product	
Protein Hydroly-sates: Marine	Proteins from the sea	Red algae, blue algae, kelp, seaweed, chlo-rella, spirullina, careegan (Irish moss)	Depends on product	
Humec-tants: Sugars	From sugar based substanc-es. Sometimes will end in "-ccharides"	Muccopolysac-charides, honey, guar gum	At bottom middle or bottom	Also called saccharides
Humec-tants: Amino Acids	Amino acids	Taurine, cys-teine, cystine, methionine	Middle	
Humec-tants: Miscella-neous		Glycerin, al-laintoin, protein hydrolysates	Depends on product	

Category 3: Additives Cheat Sheet

Group Name	Pattern/How to Identify It	Examples of It	Usual/Common Location on Label	Notes
Lubricant: Fatty materials, natural oils	Seed or bean oils, or fruit oils	Olive oil, sesame oil, walnut oil, avocado oil, apricot oil, castor oil cotton oil, sunflower oil, almond oil	Middle to bottom	Jojoba oil is technically a wax but can provide lubrication and be placed in this category.
Lubricants: Fatty materials, hydrocarbons	Made from crude oil	Mineral oil, paraffin, petrolatum, squalane	Top, Middle, Bottom	
Lubricants: fatty alcohols	"yl + alcohol"	Cetearyl alcohol, cetyl alcohol, stearyl alcohol, lauryl alcohol, myristyl alcohol	Top to middle	Lauryl alcohol is a surfactant and a solvent. Remember, some ingredients can fit in more than one category.
Lubricants: silicones	End in "-oxane", "-cone"	Cyclopentasiloxane, amodimethicone, dimethicone, dimethicone copolyol, simethicone, stearoxydimethicone	Top to middle	
Fragrance	Parfum, perfume, fragrance		Middle to bottom	Sometimes only the word fragrance or perfume is listed. For the break out of fragrance components, please refer back to the fragrance section of this book.

Category 3: Additives Cheat Sheet

Group Name	Pattern/How to Identify It	Examples of It	Usual/Common Location on Label	Notes
Preservative: Bactericide		Captan, myrstalkonium chloride	Bottom	
Preservative: Fungicide	Ends in "-linone" "one-#"	DMDM hydantoin, Disodium EDTA, tetrasodium EDTA, dimethyl ether, benzophenone-N, sodium sulfite,	Bottom	
Antimicrobial	Formaldehyde Phenolics (parabens) Alcohols Acids Chlorine derived "-chloro" Quaternary ammonium compounds "-ium +chloride" "-ium +bromide" Fatty acids	Hydontoin, urea, methyl paraben, propyl paraben, butyl paraben, methyliso-thiazolinone, methlychloroisothiazolinone, benzoic acid, sorbic acid, salicyc acid Acetamide MEA, Lauramide MIPA, Oleamide MIPA	Middle to bottom, usually bottom	
Thickener: Polysaccharide		Corn starch, pectin, cellulose, aloe vera	Middle	
Thickener: Gums		Algin, carrageenan, gum Arabic, gum tracanath, guar gum, xanthum gum	Middle to bottom	

Category 3: Additives Cheat Sheet

Group Name	Pattern/How to Identify It	Examples of It	Usual/Common Location on Label	Notes
Thickener: Resins		Balsam, benzoin gum, sandalwood oil	Middle to bottom	
Thickener: Other		Natural clays including betonite, psyllium husks, hyaluronic acid (hydrolyzed muccopolysaccharide), carbomer (acrylic acid)	Depends on the product	
pH Adjusters: Acids		Boric acid, adipic acid, citric acid, formic acid, glycolic acid, lactic acid, hydrochloric acid, phosphoric acid	Middle to bottom	
pH Adjusters: Other		Apple cider vinegar, disodium phosphate, EDTA, Sodium hydroxide	Bottom	
Viscosity Adjusters	Surfactants Others	Silica, sodium chloride (NaCL), ammonium chloride, SD alcohol, lecithin	Top to middle	Already talked about surfactants so none listed.
Vitamins		Ascorbic acid, panthenol, vitamin e, vitamin B6, biotin, vitamin A, niacinmide	Middle to bottom, usually bottom	

Category 3: Additives Cheat Sheet				
Group Name	Pattern/How to Identify It	Examples of It	Usual/Common Location on Label	Notes
Herbs, herbals, Herbal extracts, fruits	Ends in "-extract" Plants, leaves, fruit, essential oils		Middle to bottom, usually bottom	The names can be the botanical name or the plant name
Color: Natural	From natural sources	Henna, henna extract, carotene, titanium dioxide, zinc oxide, mica, betonite	Bottom, sometimes in middle, rarely at the top	If these ingredients are a specialty product such as henna by itsef or betonite by itself, then these ingredients will be listed at the top.
Color: Synthetic	From synthetic sources	FD&C, D&C, caramel, disodium EDTA copper	Lower middle to bottom	

How to Use the Cheat Sheets

Use these cheat sheets to help you better understand hair products. On the back of a product label, each ingredient is separated from the others by commas, except in the case of the last ingredient, which may be followed by a period or no punctuation mark at all.

Before you write on the Product Breakdown Worksheet, you may want to make several copies of it. It is easy to duplicate. You can even make your own. It doesn't have to be pretty, only functional! Please make copies of the Additives Breakdown Worksheet, as well. Get a couple of pencils. You'll want to be able to erase and make corrections to your work.

Find a table or a free space on the floor. Spread out your cheat sheets so you can see them all in front of you. Place your two breakdown worksheets right in front of you so that you can easily fill in with your answers.

Look at the cheat sheets and get a feel for what is on them. When you are examining a list of ingredients for any product, place each ingredient into one of the three categories on the sheets: solvent, surfactant or additive. If you are not sure in which category an ingredient fits, it is probably a surfactant. Store-bought products contain mostly surfactants. Surfactants usually have extremely long, hyphenated names.

Here are extra tips to help you:

- If the confusing ingredient appears in middle of the ingredient list and it has a long name, it is probably a surfactant.
- If the confusing ingredient appears at the end or almost at the end of the list, it is probably a preservative, most likely an anti-microbial.

Practice at home first! The first five times you will do this will take the longest. Remember, your goal is simply to categorize the ingredients, not to understand what each and every ingredient is doing. I am interested in giving you a process, not the task of memorizing a whole bunch of unrelated facts.

Once you have categorized the ingredients in a product, you can refine your process by looking up the unfamiliar ingredients online, using dictionaries or an online database of cosmetics ingredients. These are tools that support the process. I have a number of product and ingredient dictionaries. They require an investment of cash, so I suggest you get them only if you plan to continue using this process. You may determine that all this analyzing is not for you. That's okay, too!

Product Breakdown Worksheet

Solvent	Surfactant	Additive	Group Name of Additive

Additives Breakdown Worksheet

No.	Additive Used for the Product (Marked w/Check)	Additive Used for Hair (Marked w/Circle)

Action Task 1:   Write Down All the Ingredients on a Piece of Paper

Select a product to analyze. Break out the magnifying glass and get under a light. I don't care how good your eyes are, it's always challenging to try and read the ingredient labels. Write down all the ingredients and set the bottle down. Work from the paper on which you have written the ingredients.

Example: Ingredients for a shampoo

Water, sodium laureth sulfate, wheat germ-midopropyl betaine, sodium chloride, benzyl alcohol, glycerin, citric acid, burdock root extract, panthenol, hydrolyzed soy protein, grapefruit, orange.

Action Task 2:   Fill in the Product Breakdown Worksheet

Fill in the Product Breakdown Worksheet, using the cheat sheets for categories 1, 2 and 3. Don't worry if it takes you ten or fifteen minutes. This is your first time! Remember, it's about practice and familiarity.

Tip: When you identify an additive, write down the Group Name from the cheat sheet, as well. You will need to further categorize the additives.

I took one shampoo from my bathroom and filled out the Product Breakdown Worksheet. Here's what I got:

Product Breakdown Worksheet

Solvent	Surfactant	Additive	Group Name of Additive
water	sodium laureth sulfate	sodium chloride	viscosity adjuster
benzyl alcohol	wheat germ-midopyl betaine	citric acid	pH adjuster
glycerin(e)		burdock root extract	herb, herbal extract
		panthenol	vitamin
		hydrolyzed soy protein	protein hydrolysate -plant
		grapefruit	herb, herbal extract, fruit, vitamin
		orange	herb, herbal extract, fruit, vitamin

How did you do? Be patient. It took me about ten minutes to do this. Benzyl alcohol was not on my cheat sheet list. It has the word alcohol, so it follows the pattern for alcohols that are in the solvent category. Did you get tricked by the wheat germ-midopyl betaine and list it as an additive or an oil? It's a surfactant. You can tell because its name ends in the word "betaine." That puts it into the surfactant category.

Action Task 3: Use the Group Name to Help Further Categorize the Additives

Looking only at the additives category, try to identify all the additives that are not in the product to have an impact on your hair but only to support or help the product itself. These will include colors, fragrances, thickeners, preservatives, antimicrobials and pH adjusters. Write a (P) for "product" after these additives.

Next, look at the additive category again and identify the ingredients that remain. These should include conditioning agents such as proteins, humectants, lubricants, vitamins and herbal extracts. They are the ingredients that will help the surface of your hair feel smoother. Write an (H) for "hair" after these additives.

Here's what I got:

Additives Breakdown Worksheet

No.	Additive Used For the Product (Marked w/P)	Additive Used for Hair (Marked w/H)
1	sodium chloride (P)	burdock root (H)
2	citric acid (P)	hydrolyzed soy protein (H)
3	grapefruit (P)	
4	orange (P)	

How did you do? I was a bit conflicted about the grapefruit and the orange. Sometimes citrus fruits are used as weak preservatives, because of their vitamin C content. Both the grapefruit and the orange are listed last. Much of the time, the last ingredients listed in a formula are the preservatives and the color. The shampoo is not colored orange or yellow, so I assumed that these ingredients were not there for color. Hence, I considered them preservatives and marked them with a (P) to indicate that their purpose is to support the product formulation.

The burdock root and the hydrolyzed soy protein are in the product to address the needs of the hair. The soy makes this a protein shampoo. If you want a light protein treatment in your hair, this is a product you might use. But remember that shampoos are formulated so that they will rinse off the hair. Therefore, if you want lots of protein, this shampoo might not be enough. Or it might the first part of a two-step treatment: a protein shampoo followed by a protein conditioner. If you know that your hair doesn't do well with protein and you want to minimize the amount of protein you put on your hair, you might not want to use this particular shampoo.

Your decision is based upon your understanding of hair in general; your understanding of your own hair; your understanding of hair products; and your ability to put it all together. You can base your decision upon your specific, unique situation. Your question is no longer, "Is this a good shampoo?" Your question should be, "Is this a good product for me and my situation right now?" What is good for you may not work for someone else, and vice versa. Furthermore, your hair needs can and do change. You are making a decision about the product based upon your current situation. At some time in the future, you may need to change your products.

I hope you are not worn out or ready to give up. The first time is the most tedious and difficult. You are almost there!

Action Task 4: *Try to Analyze the Product Further to Determine Whether to Use It or Not*

If you go back and look at your Product Breakdown Worksheet, you will notice that this product contains three solvents and two surfactants. Water, benzyl alcohol and glycerin are solvents. In fact, benzyl alcohol can also be used as a bactericide, and glycerin can be used as a lubricant, but the charts won't get you down to that level of detail.

Once you have categorized the ingredients, you can use other resources to get more specific information about each ingredient, if you wish. But remember, the purpose of this process is not to get you to understand every single ingredient on sight. The purpose is to get you to be able to categorize the ingredients so that you have a high level understanding about what is in the formula. You can then delve into an ingredient on your own, using databases, dictionaries and other resources.

Of the two surfactants listed, one ends in the word "sulphate" and one ends in the word "betaine." If you go back to your cheat sheet, you will see that sulfate/sulphate is an anionic surfactant used for cleansing and foaming, and betaine is an amphoteric surfactant that is used to lessen the irritation of the primary surfactant, the sulfate/sulphate.

Ready for one more? Let's do one with many ingredients. And this time, let's try a conditioner.

Action Task 1:   *Write Down All the Ingredients on a Piece of Paper*

Select a product to analyze. Write down all the ingredients and set the bottle down. Work from the paper on which you have written the ingredients.

Example: Ingredients in conditioner

Water, cetyl alcohol, amodimethicone, cetearyl alcohol, cetrimonium chloride, fragrance, myristyl alcohol, behentrimonium chloride, methyl paraben, limonene, hexyl cinnamal, linalool, citric acid, citronellol, hydrolyzed animal protein, color.

Action Task 2: Fill in the Product Breakdown Worksheet

Fill in the Product Breakdown Worksheet using the category 1-3 cheat sheets.

Here's what I got:

Product Breakdown Worksheet

Solvent	Surfactant	Additive	Group Name of Additive
water	centrimonium chloride	amodimethicone	lubricant-silicone
	behentrimonium chloride	parfume	fragrance
		methyl paraben	anti-microbial
		limonene	fragrance
		Hexyl cinnamal	fragrance
		linalool	fragrance
		citric acid	pH adjuster
		citronellol	fragrance
		hydrolyzed animal protein	protein hydrolysate-animal
		color	color
		cetyl alcohol	lubricant: fatty alcohol
		cetearyl alcohol	lubricant: fatty alcohol
		myristyl alcohol	lubricant: fatty alcohol

How did you do? Again, it took me about ten minutes. Did you notice that I put all the alcohols at the bottom? The reason for this is that on my first pass, I had them listed as solvents. After I had categorized everything, I referenced the cheat sheets. That's when I saw that they are additives in the group named lubricants-silicones. Did you catch that and put them in the additives category the first time around?

I placed centrimonium chloride and behentrimonium chloride in the surfactant category. They are what are called quaternary ammonium compounds. Quaternary ammonium compounds can be used as anti-microbials. If you put them in the additives list, that would have been okay, too.

Action Task 3: Use the Group Name to Help Your Further Categorize the Additives

Looking only at the additives category, try to identify all additives that do not address the hair, but are included in the formulation to help the product itself. These would be colors, fragrances, thickeners, preservatives, antimicrobials and pH adjusters. Write (P) for "product" after these additives.

Next, go back to the additive category and identify the items that remain. These should be conditioning agents such as proteins, humectants, lubricants, vitamins and herbal extracts. They are the ingredients that will help the surface of your hair feel smoother. Write (H) for "hair" after these additives.

Here's what I got:

Additives Breakdown Worksheet

No.	Additive Used For the Product (Marked w/P)	Additive Used for Hair (Marked w/H)
1	centrimonium chloride (P)	cetyl alcohol (H)
2	behentrimonium chloride (P)	cetearyl alcohol (H)
3	parfume (P)	myristyl alcohol (H)
4	methyl paraben (P)	amodimethicone (H)
5	limonene (P)	hydrolyzed animal protein (H)
6	hexyl cinnamal (P)	
7	linalool (P)	
8	citric acid (P)	
9	citronellol (P)	
10	color (P)	

How did you do? I went ahead and listed the two surfactants as additives, since they are quaternary ammonium chloride compounds, which can be used as anti-microbials. If you put the two quaternary ammonium chlorides in the surfactant category, you can go back to the chart to find more details about them. These compounds are cationic, and they tend to be used in conditioners. Cationic surfactants tend to be used to improve the surface feel of the hair.

Action Task 4: Try to Analyze the Product Further to Determine Whether to Use It or Not

If you go back and look at your Product Breakdown Worksheet, you will notice that this product contains one solvent and two surfactants. It also breaks out the fragrance information, including not only the word "parfume" but also the components of the perfume. Why is that? That is because this product is not sold exclusively in the United States. If a product is sold in the European Union, the label must include the components of the fragrance.

Again, based upon your unique situation and needs, you are now able to determine whether this conditioner might work for you.

In Closing

Many of the surfactants you have identified may have dual roles as cleansing agents and additives. Since there are thousands of surfactants used as additives, it is best to find a dictionary or database and look up the ones you have identified, in order to determine what they are what they are actually doing for your hair.

You may think this is a lot of work. It is. Yet, if you continue to use the cheat sheet, you will become more and more familiar with it. The two columns that you need to focus on initially are the Group Name column and the Example column. These two columns should help you categorize most ingredients.

This process is a kind of alphabet. You have to do some memorization, but once you do, you will be able to use the alphabet to categorize the ingredients in hundreds and thousands of hair care products.

CHAPTER 9

Time to Confirm and Check Your Understanding

Case #1

The Situation

Josefina complains that her Afro-textured hair is dry and breaking, and she has a bald patch near her nape that wasn't there six months ago. You notice blond highlights throughout her hair. She tells you she just bought a shampoo and conditioner with the same brand name, and the first ingredients on the back of the bottles are infused seawater, dimethicone and sodium lauryl sulfate. Then she confesses that she is just starting to care for her hair again after spending eight months caring for her sick mother, who passed away six months ago.

What I Might Suggest

If Josefina has highlights, she may have damaged her hair during the coloring process, leaving it dry, brittle and porous. She didn't say whether her hair is relaxed or natural. That might be something I would ask her about.

Since her hair is breaking, I would probably suggest a protein treatment applied with dry heat, to ensure that the ingredients in the treatment bind properly to her hair. Then I would suggest that Josefina stop coloring her hair. Next, she should look for products that contain humectants, or she should add honey and glycerin, which are natural, food-grade humectants, to her conditioner. I would also suggest that she might look into doing a treatment with a product that contains amino acids, since they penetrate the hair and add moisture. I'd tell her to use steam heat to ensure that the ingredients penetrate her hair.

I would suggest that Josefina get rid of the sulfate shampoo and conditioner. If she says she just bought them and would hate to waste her money, she can soften the sulfate-infused products by diluting them. If she takes a small amount of the product and adds water, a few tablespoons of oil and maybe a bit of aloe vera, that will render the sulfates less potent and therefore possibly less damaging to her hair.

Last, I would remind Josefina that she did a wonderful thing in caring for her mother during her time of need. I would let her know that caring for someone you love can be stressful on your body and hair. I would tell her that grief, which is a form of stress, can sometimes weaken the physical systems and the hair; she needs to be gentle and patient with herself and allow herself all the time she needs to grieve. I would probably suggest that for the moment she adopt a style that will protect her hair, and would ask her to try not to manipulate her hair too much. What would you suggest?

Case #2

The Situation

Beverly is excited about her upcoming wedding. Her longtime boyfriend proposed at Christmas, and on the day after Christmas she cut her relaxed hair short all the way down to her natural texture. Here hair is now chemical and relaxer free. It's now March, and the wedding is going to take place in September, nine months after the big chop. Beverly is considering wearing her hair either in a fierce twist-out or in a straight, ironed-flat style for her wedding day. Her hair looks healthy. The hair has grown three inches since the big chop.

Beverly tells you that if she wears twists on her wedding day, she wants the twists to hang thick and long past her shoulders; she hopes to gain 18 inches of growth by then. With her eyes aglow, she shows you her shampoo and says, "I bought this great product to try to get three inches of growth every month. That should put me at the length I want for September." The key ingredient in the product is a patented blend called "Grow Hair Fast." She then says that she blow dries her hair, and in order to help it grow faster and look longer she uses a flat iron every two days to stretch out the length. Her reason for this is twofold: she wants to simulate what her hair will look like in September, and she hopes the heat will soften some of her brittle, split ends. She confides that she has bad hair, and whether it's twist-ed or straightened on the big day, she doesn't think it will photograph nicely.

What I Might Suggest

Although the excitement of planning a wedding can be euphoric, it can create a tremendous amount of stress, too. I would mention this and remind Beverly to focus on herself. I'd suggest that she try to manage the stress consciously as she plans her day of a lifetime.

The great thing about Beverly is that she knows what her goal is: she wants to gain length. But Beverly is not familiar with the nature of the human hair fiber, which grows approximately one-half inch per month. Her lack of knowledge is allowing her to expect that she will gain three inches of growth every month over the six months from April to September. Beverly's lack of knowledge may cause her tremendous disappointment.

Beverly has selected her product in accordance with her goal, but the promises made by the product should not be the only thing on which she bases her decision. I would ask her for the product ingredients. You really can't afford to use only secret ingredients on your precious hair. Beverly has relied upon marketing, and she doesn't know what's in the "Grow Fast" blend contained in the product. She seems to be hoping for a magical result from this product.

I would congratulate Beverly on wanting to have the best hair possible for her day, and I'd tell her that a twist-out style is always gorgeous in healthy hair. Then I would address her excessive use of heat. Heat drying your hair brings it quickly to dryness. Dry hair tends to break, and breaking hair does not retain length. I'd tell Beverly that using so much heat so frequently will produce results contrary to her desired goals. I would suggest that she stop applying heat and use a moisture treatment followed by a deep protein treatment. I would teach her how to protect and seal the ends of her hair to help soften them. If she decides to wear her hair heat-pressed on the day of her wedding, I would suggest that she use a reconstructor for the temporary repair of split ends. This will give her ends a silky appearance and will help the straightened hair to photograph well. If she decides to wear twists, I would suggest that she select a shampoo with humectants and lots of conditioning agents. Natural Afro-textured hair thrives on moisture, and humectant-infused products will keep the moisture locked into her twists.

The last point I would address would be the "bad hair" comment. I would remind Beverly that healthy hair is beautiful. There is no such thing as bad hair; there is only the lack of knowledge and skill that makes so many women unable to manage their hair. What would you suggest?

Case #3

The Situation

Rachel is totally bald around her hairline and on the entire left side of her head. She lifts her weave, shows you the thin, fine hair underneath and tells you that her weave can no longer be glued to this area because there is no more hair left. Rachel says she goes to an internationally famous weave specialist, and if he can't stop her breakage, the problem must be her hair. She says she will probably end up bald, but luckily her stylist makes a line of really cute wigs and at least she'll be able to wear one of those. She laughs, but you can tell that she is uncomfortable and sad about her hair.

What I Might Suggest

I would tell Rachel that there are many gifted stylists out there who can create great styles and keep hair healthy. I would gently let her know that balding hairlines and thin or missing hair are signs that the hair is not healthy. Rachel's hair is weakened and tremendously damaged. I would suggest that she stop getting glued-on weaves. I would also suggest that she take a break from relaxers for at least six months. I would encourage her to select a wig she can use while giving her hair a rest. I would explain how to keep her new growth moist, softened and nourished.

I would try to help Rachel set reasonable expectations. I'd let her know that her hair has been over-processed, and so it is likely that it will begin to break from the ends up. If hair is not over-processed, you can go for several months or a year without a touch-up or having relaxer chemical applied to the new growth, and have minimal breakage, but in order to achieve this you must know how to care for your hair, how to detangle it and style it using low manipulation, and you must have products that you know work for you.

I would let Rachel know that weaves and wigs can be used to support healthy hair, but you must care for the hair underneath them. I would suggest that although sew-in weaves are not as damaging as glued-on hair, even sew-in weaves would not be best for her right now because she needs to have very little stress or weight placed on her hair. What would you suggest?

Case #4

The Situation

Shawndra tells you that for the last five weeks her scalp has been itching and flaking so much that now it is inflamed. You can see that she has open and infected sores on her scalp. Shawndra has beautiful hair that is thick and full with perfect ends, and she wears it in a huge Afro, but her scalp is oozing and painful. She is embarrassed by the state of her scalp. She says she has tried every dandruff shampoo on the market and is at her wits' end. She is thinking about shaving her head, but doesn't want to lose the magnificent Afro she has cultivated over the last two years.

Shawndra tells you that she managed her company's Paris office for a month, and she got braids with hair extensions because she thought it would be an easy-to-manage style that would allow her to focus on her career. She selected synthetic hair extensions because they matched her hair color the best, and she left the braids in for the entire month she was in Paris. She has been back for about a week, and although she has removed the extensions, the problem on her scalp has gotten worse. She assumes that living abroad and speaking only in French every day was stressful. This stress impacted her body and perhaps it was the stress that caused her scalp to itch. She is thinking about getting some more braids so that her scalp can breathe. She still has some synthetic hair left over, and she could get a friend to help her put in more extensions.

What I Might Suggest

Living and working abroad can be stressful, even when the situation is fun and exciting. I would ask Shawndra if she has any other skin irritations on the rest of her body. If she does not, I would conclude that it was probably not the water in her Paris apartment that caused the problem. Once I eliminated that, I would ask if she has ever had a similar experience of itching and inflammation. If she has not, I would look for what has changed in her life. First I would focus on the most recent five weeks. In Shawndra's case, she had the life-changing event of moving to France. The other thing Shawndra did in the last five weeks was get hair extensions for the first time. She's mentioned that the hair extensions were synthetic and that her scalp started to itch while she was in Paris. This coincides with the time she got the extensions. Although she has removed the extensions, the itching remains. This does not mean that it wasn't the hair that caused the itching. If something irritates your body, the reaction may not go away as soon as you remove the irritating substance. The scalp and body absorb irritants, and the body then reacts to remove them, in this case by creating itching and inflammation.

I would suggest that Shawndra not place any more extensions, synthetic or otherwise, in her gorgeous hair. I would encourage her to braid her hair gently so that the scalp can be exposed and examined, and then to go see a dermatologist immediately and follow his or her instructions. I would encourage Shawndra to make sure the dermatologist is knowledgeable about these kinds of situations. You can't assume that just because someone is a stylist, he or she will focus on the health of your hair, and in the same way you can't assume that just because someone is a doctor, he or she will be able to help you resolve your situation. The worst thing to encounter when experiencing hair issues is an insensitive doctor who couldn't care less about your health concerns. What would you suggest for Shawndra?

Case #5

The Situation

Monique tells you her hair is thin and fine, and she doesn't know what she wants to do with it. She says she is looking for a product to make her hair as thick as her best friend's hair. She can't understand why she doesn't gain any length, because she regularly cuts off one or two inches of hair every other month to avoid split ends. She does this because she has always heard that hair that didn't have split ends was healthy. She also mentions that she's heard that crushing birth control pills and putting them in your shampoo makes your hair grow faster.

What I Might Suggest

I would suggest that Monique not use crushed birth control pills, no matter what someone has claimed they have done for their hair. Birth control pills are bioactive. This means that the hormones they contain can affect the internal physical systems and organs, even if they are just put on your hair. Using them indiscriminately without being under a doctor's care can create problems you can't afford. African-American women have high levels of fibroid tumors; furthermore, although African-American women as a group do not have the highest incidence of breast cancer, more African-American women die from breast cancer than our sisters who are not of African-American descent. Abnormal production of the hormone estrogen is involved in the development of both fibroids and breast cancer.

I would suggest that Monique learn more about the hair and scalp. Much of her product selection has been based on what she has heard. It is okay to investigate products because of what you've heard, but this is not a good basis for your final decisions.

I would encourage Monique to determine what her hair goals are. She needs to figure out what she wants to accomplish with her hair. I would ask her to define her idea of beautiful hair. I would encourage her to get to know her hair, not just the aspects of it she perceives to be negative or unattractive but the positive aspects, as well. I would then suggest that she identify some of the challenges of her hair. She mentioned that it was always thin and limp. I would explain that if you keep the ends of your hair even, it looks thicker, but you can't do anything to make naturally thin hair thicker. I would ask Monique to write down her discoveries and document her hair with pictures.

Finally, I would encourage Monique to look at how she cares for her hair. How does she style it? What products does she use? What are the ingredients in her products? Then I would volunteer to sit with her and try to put it all together.

In essence, I would walk Monique through the Hair Care Products 101 Four-Step Process. That would empower her to make her own informed choices about her hair and its care. I'd tell her to stop relying on what she's heard and stop looking at products or actions in isolation. She should find out what the product claims to do, determine whether that claim can support her in reaching the goals she has identified or resolving her challenge, and then analyze the product before making her decision. Process-based methods are more effective than the "I heard" method. I would remind her always to look at her entire situation and what she wants to accomplish. What would you suggest?

Some Encouraging Final Words

When you are planning to purchase a store-bought product, you must know what your problem or challenge is, examine why you have the problem, and look for the products to help you resolve it. This will help you have realistic expectations about what the product can do for you. The money and disappointment you save will make this process invaluable.

Using the Four-Step Hair Products 101 Process, you can select products based on your knowledge of the hair fiber in general, your own unique hair needs and goals, and what products are formulated to do. You can know what's in the bottle by knowing what's on the bottle.

Now, please go back and look over the ingredients in that $150 product I mentioned at the beginning of the book. Although you may not understand the ingredients completely, you will have an idea of what they are and what they are meant to do. Although you won't know every single thing that is in the product, most of those ingredients will be familiar enough that you will be able to categorize them. If you can do that, I have accomplished what I set out to do.

Never forget that it's all about practice and familiarity. You are truly in control of which products you select. Wield your power and money wisely!

References

Alexander, Peter and Hudson, Robert F., *Wool Its Chemistry and Physics.* Chapman and Hall LTD, London. 1963

Baumann, Leslie. *Cosmetic Dermatology: Principles and Practices,* Second Edition.McGraw-Hill Professional, New York. 2009

Goddard, Desmond, E. and Gruber, James V., *Principles of Polymer Science and Technology in Cosmetics and Personal Care,* Marcel Dekker, Inc. 1999

Hunting, Anthony, *Encyclopedia of Conditioning Rinse Ingredients,* Micelle Press, England. 2004

Hunting, Anthony, *Encyclopedia of Shampoo Ingredients,* Micelle Press, England. 1983

Kamath, Y. K., Hornby, Sidney B., Weigman, H, D. "Mechanical and Fractographic Behavior of Negroid Hair." *Journal of Cosmetic Chemistry,* 35, 21-43 (January/February 1984).

Robbins, C.R., Bahl, M.K. "Analysis of Hair by Electron Spectroscopy for Chemical Analysis." *Journal of Cosmetic Chemistry,* 35, 379-390 (December 1984).

Robbins, Clarence R. *Chemical and Physical Behavior of Human Hair,* Springer, New York. 2002

Schueller, Randy and Romanowski, Perry, *Conditioning Agents for Hair and Skin,* Marcel Dekker, Inc., New York. 1999

Swift, Alan J., *Cosmetic Science Monographs* No. 1 "Fundamentals of Human Hair Science," Micelle Press, England. 1997

Swift, Alan J. "Mechanism of Split End Formation in Human Head Hair." *Journal of Cosmetic Chemistry,* 48, 123-126 (March/April 1997).

www.ingramcontent.com/pod-product-compliance
Lightning Source LLC
Chambersburg PA
CBHW072200270326
41930CB00011B/2496